Anna Mathur is a mother of three and an experienced psychotherapist accredited by the British Association for Psychotherapy and Counselling. She is passionate about taking therapy out of the therapy room, empowering people to utilise simple techniques that will help them reframe the way that they think. The most pertinent thing about the way she communicates isn't the letters after her name, but the way in which she weaves her own experience through her writing.

Anna Mathur

MIND
Over
MOTHER

Every mum's guide to worry
and anxiety in the first year

piatkus

PIATKUS

First published in Great Britain in 2020 by Piatkus

3 5 7 9 10 8 6 4

A CIP catalogue record for this book
is available from the British Library.

ISBN 978-0-349-42542-9

Typeset in Bembo by M Rules
Printed and bound in Great Britain by Clays Ltd, Elcograf S.p.A.

Papers used by Piatkus are from well-managed forests
and other responsible sources.

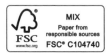

Piatkus
An imprint of
Little, Brown Book Group
Carmelite House
50 Victoria Embankment
London EC4Y 0DZ

An Hachette UK Company
www.hachette.co.uk

www.improvementzone.co.uk

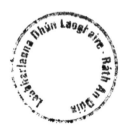

For Tarun and Mum.
Your faithfulness and cheerleading are the wind in my sails.
And for my kids who through their love have ushered me
to become myself.

Contents

Introduction

Anxiety didn't just hit me like a broken dam. It chipped away like a small hammer, slowly sending hairline fractures throughout the core of who I knew myself to be, both as an individual and as a mother. The increasing fear cracked my smile at its corners and splintered my peace.

And then, in a moment of sharp clarity, I realised that I couldn't remember the last time I had gone to sleep peacefully. I only knew exhaustion provoked by whirlwinds of overthinking. I couldn't remember the last time I'd treated myself with kindness, I knew only self-criticism. And I couldn't remember the last time I felt love for my children that hadn't been marred by a sharp fear of loss.

It took strength to fight against the negative things I had grown to believe about myself. It took courage to be honest about my reality. But it was the best and strongest thing I've ever done. It was the end and the beginning of so much. And that journey is the fuel for my writing this book.

Anxiety no longer robs me of myself. And it need not rob you either.

Why I've written this book for you

I'm Anna, a psychotherapist and a mum of three. I'm a perfectionist and a people-pleaser in ongoing recovery, with a wild penchant for Instagram, an increasing tolerance of life's chaos, and a rocky relationship with baking.

I've been itching to write this book for you for a while. It's the book I wish I'd had on my bedside table when I had my first baby. It would have undoubtedly changed my experience of motherhood. Anxiety impacts us mums more than it needs to. It takes up more headspace than it deserves. It can prevent us from making certain decisions or speaking out about our feelings, wants and needs.

I have written this book so that you can claim some of that precious headspace back. So that less of life will be tainted by the whisper of the 'what ifs'. You'll learn a lot about yourself amidst these pages. You'll gain a deeper understanding of anxiety and be armed with techniques and tips to help.

This is an investment, because these approaches won't just benefit your experience of motherhood, you can call upon them for the rest of your life. I love to imagine this book will be well thumbed, scribbled in and splattered with life. I'm passionate about the words that fill these pages because I've lived them. I've not only seen these concepts change the lives of my clients, they've also changed mine.

My journey to motherhood

My first baby, Oscar, was a dark-haired dreamboat. I felt an overwhelming love as soon as I met him. It was like a wave that drenched my heart and caused it to double in size within moments. That first year was generally a happy one, navigating life as a first-time mum, filled with play dates, café cake, routine chat, mutual sleep moans and enough coffee to float a ship.

By the time Oscar blew out (read: 'liberally spat over') his first birthday cake candles, I was pregnant again. I knew it because my hormones were rife and I had to swallow down many argumentative quips that threatened to pop out at my husband, as we celebrated with family.

And there was the blue line a week later. I took the test at 5 a.m. (early pregnancy hormones have me wired at 5 a.m. and eyeing up the bed at 5 p.m.). I left it on the toilet lid for my husband to find when he went in for his 6 a.m., pre-commute shower. Romantic.

Then began a very different journey, one of extreme morning sickness, appendicitis (for me), tongue-ties (apparently, they can reattach), undiagnosed silent reflux, bonding issues, chronic sleep deprivation, and stifling postnatal anxiety and depression. I'll speak of this in different ways throughout the book. That year had me digging down to depths of myself I hadn't seen before, and I discovered a strength I had never had to use before either. I didn't feel strong, in fact I felt incredibly stuck, and weak, and lost. But I must have been strong. It's undeniable. Because I'm here to tell the tale.

And I did it again. It took me a while to consider having another baby. We'd always dreamt of three, until that point. I had to really put things into place before going through the process of trying for a third, and all of those are here, in this book.

I had to increase the self-care (in a non-cheesy have-a-lovely-bubble-bath way), address my rather stern internal chatter and speak more about my feelings.

Some babies are harder than others. But also, we all have different internal challenges and histories that impact our experiences.

I had to put my dangerous 'super-mum' aspiration well and truly to bed. Those things saved me. They've saved me over and over as I've had to revisit them, because old habits die hard.

Anyway, along came Florence. Baby number three and a balm to the trauma of my previous post-natal experience. I'm only now realising quite how different babies can be, and how their challenges challenge us. I had three different babies and three utterly different journeys, and a map for none. I'm hoping that what I've learnt in the lecture theatres, the consulting rooms, and my own personal experience will help provide a map for you.

Becoming a therapist

After studying for a degree in Social Psychology, I gained a master's degree in Psychotherapy and Counselling at Regent's University London. There I began my journey to becoming an accredited psychotherapist with the British Association for Counselling and Psychotherapy.

Before we did the classic we're-having-a baby-so-let's-move-out-of-the-city-because-we-can barely-afford-a-studio-flat, I'd been living in London working as a psychotherapist in private practices and in GP surgeries. I would sit with individuals weekly, from anything between six weeks, to three years. We'd do quick work, deep work, 'tell me about your relationship with your father' work. I loved it.

We moved out of London one spring weekend, with a groaning rent-a-van and an eight-week-old secret in my belly (although it was obvious if you caught a glimpse of my green-tinged face). For a while I commuted into London to see my existing clients, but I slowly moved my practice locally. I now see clients in the comfort of my own home, inviting them to sit on my squishy blue sofa.

I once heard that when you train as a therapist, you get the therapy you need. I trained as a therapist because I wanted to help people untangle their minds, but really, mine needed a good lot of untangling too. In fact, I'll be untangling my mind and thoughts in some form forever. But I'm increasingly OK with that.

Whilst I have the skills to help others, I cannot be my very own one-woman support network. You cannot be your one-woman support network either, regardless of how much knowledge, experience and self-awareness you have. Knowledge prepares, equips and allows us to change and shift things, but it doesn't prevent. In a way, whilst I've experienced some challenging twists and turns in the roller-coaster that is motherhood, I am kind of grateful for them.

They ignited the fire of passion in my belly for postnatal mental health.

I love working with people who have anxiety because ultimately, with the right guidance and insight, tips and tools, their lives can change pretty darn quickly. I love the light-bulb moments that occur when people make new connections between past and present, and emotion and action. Something amazing happens when clients realise they aren't the only ones thinking or feeling as they do. The embarrassment and shame begin to get chipped away. I consider it an immense honour to be part of that process.

Being the therapist in therapy

Training as a therapist came with the requirement of experiencing therapy. I obligingly found a therapist, considering it as a box-ticking exercise. Because, you know, I actually wanted to help other people. I myself was fine thank you very much.

It turned out, therapy was exactly what I needed. It was a chance to recognise my own messy bits; it was time to peek into the darker corners of my mind. Therapy has taught me that my own mental health challenges don't discount me from being a good therapist.

The more I work on my own challenges, the more I acknowledge them and don't fear them, the more useful a therapist I am. That is why you'll read some of my own experiences woven throughout this book.

This is motherhood

I've sat with hundreds of mums over my ten years as a therapist, and spoken with thousands through my work on social media. There's an epidemic of mum-guilt, a wave of worry about the big and the small things. There's a cultural drive to need to please everyone around us, a concern that we are 'doing the right thing'.

We fear putting a foot wrong, but we are so bombarded by advice from all angles that we have lost touch with our own sense of what's right for *us*. We're encouraged to constantly compare ourselves to others as a measure of how well we're doing, or not.

I'd be lying if I said you would never worry or feel anxious as a mum on completing this book. No, anxiety will still knock at your door. However, I hope it will be less likely to rule your life, decisions and moods.

We're going to cut out the noise. We're going to bring the focus back to you. We're going to address the worry that has become so accepted as part of motherhood. We're going to smash some taboos and get you to the point where you feel equipped and grounded on this rollercoaster ride that is motherhood.

There is a new level of openness surrounding motherhood. However, I don't believe we should stop there. There's so much more to it than laughing about 'mum fails' and shrugging off our 'mum guilt' as a way of saying 'hey, that's part of the job description', as if it's an inevitability.

Because it doesn't need to be. There's more.

And that's what I'm here to tell you.

How you can make the most out of this book

Journaling

Should you want to do them, at the end of each chapter you'll find a few guided journal questions for you to answer. These questions make the words of the text personal to you.

I'll throw my hands up and say I'm no journaler. I have some old, dog-eared journals packed with scrawled thoughts from years ago, back when I had headspace and time to laze in bed and was less likely to wake up to find the imprint of a pen on my hip. These days, if I'm to jot any thoughts down, I like it to be concise and guided.

Writing things down helps the brain regulate emotion.

Consider treating yourself to a new journal. Whether you quickly jot down single sentences or find yourself writing reams of thoughts, that's totally fine. There's no right or wrong way. But I will encourage you, because writing things down helps the brain regulate emotion in a different way to speaking or thinking about it.

If you don't feel like journaling, maybe read the questions through anyway and consider them for a moment. You may be surprised at a mini breakthrough or light-bulb moment that follows.

Tips

There are a whole wealth of practical tips to help with your anxiety coming up in Chapter 11. But in the meantime, I've added a suggestion to each chapter for those who want to try some techniques to help along the way.

Mantras

I've written a mantra for you in each chapter. They are small sentences that you can repeat to yourself whenever you feel you need some motivation or support. I find them really helpful and you might too.

Chapter 1

Challenging your 'normal'

Mantra: I give myself permission to take things slowly.

It doesn't matter whether you have 'anxiety' written on your doctor's notes or not, it's worth addressing. It may be that anxiety only has the smallest effect on your life or is something that comes in waves. Perhaps you've never once web-searched 'can sleep deprivation actually kill you?', but maybe you've dropped a bottle of milk and cursed yourself, or felt you were failing at this motherhood lark.

Whether you were handed this book by a friend or purchased it during a night-feed internet search spree, I'm glad you have it. I'm going to tell you how it all works, and why I know that diving into these pages is going to be such a worthy investment of your precious time.

We all feel anxious sometimes

In researching this book, I asked many mums whether they'd describe themselves as anxious or if they'd experienced anxious thoughts. Many replied saying they didn't, but they often felt worried. However, on hearing from me some examples of anxious thoughts, every single mother agreed that they experienced anxiety to some level, with varying effects on their life.

Not everyone relates to the word 'anxiety', but I'm going to put something out there ...

We all feel anxious sometimes.

There is a difference between worry and anxiety. In a nutshell, worry tends to be initiated by real-life events, and might prompt you to do something. It might be that you're worried about being late, so you leave earlier. Or you're worried about a physical issue, so you book a doctor's appointment. You're able to think about your concern rationally, and once the event has passed, the worry subsides. Anxiety, however, feels harder to control and is more likely to impact your quality of life. It may come with physical symptoms and often includes cycles of overthinking. If you'd like to look at the difference between worry and anxiety in more detail, turn to pages 24–5.

Worry can progress into anxiety. This is so easily done when worry remains unchecked, and tired or compromised minds struggle to keep things rational. There is no doubt that you'll worry from time to time, or from moment to moment. Anxiety is worth addressing, regardless of how much it impacts you. We always benefit from understanding it more, and practising some simple techniques that will help lessen the anxiety. We shouldn't allow it the power to impact our enjoyment of life, ourselves and motherhood.

Changing your 'normal'

The majority of us aren't that kind to ourselves in the secret world of our heads, which only fuels this heightened sense of worry. We have a habit of berating ourselves like a strict teacher. We can find it hard to accept the support that others offer us and fear being a burden because our culture lauds the 'I've got this' supermum ideal.

In its true form, anxiety is a natural human state, and we're going to look at many facets of it that will be impacting your life. From the way you talk to yourself, to tips and tools to ground yourself in those exhausted moments when you feel like You. Just. Can't. Do. This. (But you can, because you do, over and over.) Whilst anxiety might feel like it's your 'normal', it doesn't need to be.

Just because anxiety might feel like it's your 'normal', it doesn't need to be.

This book is laced with the voices of other mums that will tell you you're not alone or mad. Whether your anxiety is bubbling under the surface of your smile, creeping up on you when you're tired, or holding you hostage, I've written this for you.

I'm going to make this book worth your energy

From one mother to another, I know this isn't a small deal for you. It takes a lot of courage to address these things, and energy too, of which I know you probably don't have in abundance right now.

However, I promise you it's such a worthwhile invest-ment of the scraps of energy you do have. Read a few lines here and there; tuck it under your favourite squishy seat of the sofa. By the end, I hope you'll feel more able to enjoy the happy moments and find yourself more equipped for the tougher ones. Your head will be a more peaceful place to be and your internal chatter hopefully kinder.

I believe you will find this book helpful, no matter how your anxiety presents itself. I'm going to encourage you to gently challenge the thoughts that have been impacting your confidence, your resources to cope. We're going to address the things that have been holding you back from moving forward. We'll go on a tour of many aspects of anxiety. I will help you reframe and reclaim your authority back from its familiar grasp, so that you can begin to thrive in your role as mother.

Take it at your own pace

If I ask one thing of you, it's that you are kind to yourself as you read this book. It's a brave thing to address your thoughts; especially when sleep deprived and having gone through the biggest life shift any woman can go through.

I must admit, I have an inbuilt 'go hard or go home' attitude. I try to tackle everything at 110 per cent and then fizzle out 60 per cent of the way through and leave things to gather dust. I have a whole collection of crochet books on the shelf, but I couldn't get beyond a wonky square. I should probably take them to the charity shop.

I have to fight that attitude often. Slow and steady really

does win the race. Don't feel you have to storm through this book answering every question and writing reams of journal notes. Actually, *don't* storm through it. Instead, give yourself permission to take it easy and go as slowly as you need to.

When addressing anxiety, there's no rush. Slow and steady wins the race.

There simply is no wrong way! Turn down a corner mid-chapter or shut it mid-sentence – be kind to yourself. Slow and steady.

Further support

The advice and techniques given within this book are not intended to replace or conflict with advice given by your doctor or healthcare professional.

If while reading you realise that certain experiences you've had might be fuelling some of your negative thoughts, or you recognise that some of your thought patterns are rooted in a specific event, I recommend that you explore the option of therapy.

My favourite online resource for finding a therapist is the Counselling Directory, otherwise your doctor may be able to refer you to a local service. You might like to take some of your notes to discuss with a therapist or friend. If you need some extra support or input, please don't push through it alone.

Later on in the book I look at vulnerability and how important it is for good mental health, but you can always flick forward to that chapter (see page 190) should you need the encouragement.

Your expectations about the book

Dealing with our thoughts can sometimes feel a bit time consuming and tiring, because we're met with thousands upon thousands of thoughts every day.

Addressing negative thought patterns is such a worthy investment because they can easily fill your mind, suck joy out of situations, create unease and creep into your dreams. If you can cope with these thoughts day in, day out as you establish life as a mum to a new babe, then that takes a certain kind of strength.

You're already stronger than you think you are, regardless of what you believe. You've mustered the strength to make it this far, despite the internal rollercoaster, and therefore, with the right support, you'll have the strength to begin to implement tools that will help.

I'm writing not purely as a psychotherapist but as a mum who is emerging fresh (ha! Who am I kidding? I'm slightly bedraggled but with a full heart) from my third postnatal period. The words I am going to share with you are an amalgamation of my years of psychotherapy training and client work with mums. However, most importantly of all, these concepts, tools and insights have undoubtedly changed my life, and the way that I feel on a daily basis. I experienced anxiety before being a mother, but motherhood certainly kicked it up to a whole new level.

Addressing the way we think isn't a linear process and sometimes you may feel as though you're taking two steps back and one step forward, or not moving at all. Don't forget, you're likely tired and navigating the motherhood juggle, so your ability to rationalise every tricky thought that skips through your mind is going to be challenged. Extra self-kindness is necessary.

It's entirely natural to feel as if you're doing some kind of mental salsa dance, moving forward and backward with tentative toes. Lots of anxiety-fuelled behaviours and thought patterns have an ingrained, habitual element. (I use the word 'habitual' quite a lot in this book to describe behaviours and ways of thinking that have become a habit. They often feel quite repetitive and a bit like a reflex.)

It sure sounds like a bit of work, right? But I want to reassure you that this is the best investment of any remaining dregs of your energy right now. This is about *you* and giving yourself the opportunity to enjoy your motherhood journey as best you can.

Perhaps choose to replace a moment's mindless scrolling with reading some of this book. You'd be surprised how much mental energy is used whizzing through shiny photos that often poke at that slightly vulnerable spot where you don't feel quite 'enough'. This is a far better use of those ten minutes, and will help you to realise quite how 'enough' you are.

Don't go it alone

As you read, consider who you might like to speak to
should it raise some topics for further discussion. It might
be a partner or a friend from your antenatal group, a
therapist or family member, but tell someone who knows
you, and who has in the past been supportive, kind and
empathetic. I want you to have at least one person who
can be available for you if you need to discuss anything in
further depth.

This is for you

Maybe you identify with having had anxiety for years.
Perhaps it pounced on you as you saw the blue lines on your
pregnancy test, or that moment you heard the first cry in
the delivery room.

Whatever journey has led you to pick up this book, I've
written it for you.

I'm glad you're here.

Top Tip

Treat yourself to a new journal. Scribble, draw,
write single words or essays. Make it your own.

JOURNAL POINTS

- How do you feel about opening this book? What would you like to achieve?
- Do you believe we are all anxious?
- Can you identify any themes with your anxiety? Any particular fears or focuses?
- If you wanted to chat through any element of this book with someone, who would you choose?

Chapter 2

Anxiety. Moving from chilled to frozen

Mantra: *I am not my thoughts.*

It seems to have become culturally acceptable to spend our lives teetering back and forth between worry and anxiety. As mothers, we tend to quickly demote all the things that might help us feel more relaxed and grounded. It takes more time and effort to schedule in some space, to focus on a breathing exercise, to call a friend or to go for a walk than it takes to fall back on our habit of ruminating. Habits are habits because they are so much easier to engage in, regardless of how unhelpful they are.

It seems to have become culturally acceptable to spend our lives teetering back and forth between worry and anxiety.

And because it has become culturally acceptable, we forget that we can do something to change it and make things better for ourselves. Anxiety is the thief that steals precious headspace, impacting our peace and enjoyment of motherhood. To be able to change this, we must first get down to the bones of anxiety. And that's what we're about to do.

Drawing the line

I imagine anxiety sitting on a line amidst other emotional states. I have drawn it out, so we can explore this in a little more detail.

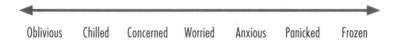

| Oblivious | Chilled | Concerned | Worried | Anxious | Panicked | Frozen |

Imagine yourself on this line as a colourful marble. You are continuously moving up and down this line. It might feel like you settle in one place for a while, but you're never there for long – your body and mind simply can't maintain any single state constantly.

We're all here because we generally spend more time towards the right end of the scale, but don't be seduced into thinking that all is fine and dandy down the other end. Being at either end has repercussions. Both have their positives and negatives. The most mentally and physically healthy place to spend the majority of our time is somewhere near the middle, and that's what we're working towards.

Oblivious

At one end of the scale sits 'oblivious'. This is when you are so immersed in something that you lack any consciousness of risk. You've become oblivious to the repercussions of your own actions and the dangers around you. Imagine you are so absorbed in painting, or a piece of music, that you don't even hear people calling your name. It's like you've merged into whatever you are doing. However, if you remain in this unaware state for an extended amount of time, it makes you very vulnerable. It's similar to how being very drunk or drugged can cause people to act recklessly and dangerously, as risk and repercussions aren't considered. Your thinking and actions are far from rational.

> *When I'm painting, it's like the world is totally and utterly shut out. I don't even recognise when I'm hungry or if someone is calling for me. It's like all of my senses are totally engaged in what I'm doing. It's amazing but it feels like a harsh crash back down to earth when I snap out of it.*
>
> Chen

Chilled

Rationality has crept in. You're really relaxed and aware of where you are and what's going on around you but you feel quite disconnected from it. It's like that feeling of being on the ultimate holiday. You're aware of your responsibilities and the pull of different elements of your life that are kind of carrying on regardless without you. But you don't feel worried about whether the cat has been fed by your neighbour or the contents of the unopened mail on your doormat.

Staying in that chilled state would be bliss, like lying in a bath of bubbles forever. But realistically, the water cools, your fingers get wrinkly. Then the phone rings. Your time in the tub has to end and you know it. Real life is calling you and needs you back. But you love it whilst it lasts.

Being relaxed is a grounding place to be but it sure can take practice and effort to get there and stay there. You acknowledge thoughts of the past and the future but you don't hold onto them. They slip through your hands like sand, and you realise that the only real living to be done is here. Where you are.

The last time I felt really relaxed was on Sunday. I'd had lunch with my family, we all felt lazy and full and content. I didn't feel worried about going to work on Monday or catching up on emails. It felt good.

Pippa

Concerned

You are aware of an issue but you aren't particularly emotionally invested in it. You are able to consider it when you need to or choose to and it doesn't prompt a strong emotional or physical response. You are thinking rationally, you are aware of risk but not fearful of it.

Concern tends to be rooted in real circumstances. It's a temporary state that comes and goes as circumstances arise and pass. It can actually be quite motivating, often leading to problem solving and action being taken. You might have a concern about making an appointment on time but you channel it into being organised and paying closer attention to the time. Then when the appointment is met, the concern subsides.

Perhaps you hear a sad story. A friend tells you something that happened to a friend of theirs that you don't know. You feel concerned but you don't instantly put yourself in the situation and imagine it happening to you or someone you love. You feel a bit separate from it. It's sad but it's not happening to you, it may never happen to you.

> *My friend's nan has cancer. Don't get me wrong, I feel for her family and I really don't mind her talking to me about it. It's sad for them and I care for my friend. If I'm totally honest, I don't feel that emotional myself because she's old and it's like the natural progression of life.*

Anonymous

Worried

You are worried. Something is starting to linger in your mind and you're chewing on it like a piece of gum. Rationality is wavering, dependent on how long you spend chewing. You feel more emotionally invested in the situation and it's taking up more headspace.

Your child has a temperature and whilst you know rationally that it's likely to be a commonplace virus, you read an article about sepsis recently and the symptom list keeps popping into your mind. You switch between re-assuring yourself that all will be OK to feeling pangs of fear that it isn't. You are able to make a plan. You'll monitor the temperature and administer paracetamol. If it hasn't gone down by a set time, you'll seek some advice. You are rational and emotionally engaged but your marble is being nudged between worry and anxiety depending on how grounded you're feeling in any moment.

My brain quite likes a good old worry. It doesn't always bother me that much. I tend to reassure myself with statistics or tell myself that what I'm worried about is probably going to be fine. Unless it switches on at night and I can't stop thinking about whatever it is. Then I can't sleep because it steps up a level and I feel all revved up.

Dominique

Anxiety

The small worry has become an increasingly loud storm in your mind. The more you think about it, the more your heart rate starts to increase, and the less you are able to think about it rationally. You feel restless because these thoughts are telling your body that there is a threat. You feel a physical reaction of some level, because your nervous system is responding to fear and preparing you to react.

Your thoughts are more intense and fixated on the issue or situation. If you unpick them, you'll likely discover that your thoughts are fear-based. You find it hard to keep this kind of thinking at bay as it creeps into your thoughts and maybe your dreams.

Anxiety includes more mental imagery. It's like making up bad stories about what might happen. As you replay them, it can lead to emotional distress. It saps your ability to experience joy and consumes an increasing amount of headspace. You may begin to engage in certain behaviours to try to regain a sense of safety.

You try hard to grasp the rational voice to reassure yourself. Maybe you call a friend or do a breathing exercise to calm your body and mind. If you catch yourself as the storm begins to pick up speed, this is easier to do. But as anxiety increases and moves more towards panic, grounding yourself becomes more challenging.

Sometimes I get a thought and then it really won't go away. It starts to stress me out and I can't stop thinking about it. It's typically based on something bad happening and the more I think about it, the more convinced I am and the harder it is to tell myself it's going to be OK. My chest feels heavier and heavier if that makes sense.

Anonymous

Panic

When you panic, it can feel like things are spiralling. The rational mind sounds like a far-away, blurred echo. You feel like you're on a malfunctioning rollercoaster that won't stop. You want to get off but the attendant isn't paying attention. It feels intense and scary.

Your nervous system is fuelling your body in order to fight or escape the trigger and regain a sense of safety. Your body is under stress and you feel increasing physical symptoms such as rapid heart and breathing rates. You may experience a panic attack if you aren't able to find a way to calm your breathing and bring your mind back into the present.

Your feelings will be impacting the decisions you are making. Your actions and reactions are designed to pro-tect you. You might remove yourself from the situation as quickly as you can without thinking much about any social or physical consequences.

Panic is a heightened physical state and your body can't physically sustain it for long. Everything is firing on full cylinders in order to protect your life, but it takes a lot of energy to maintain, which is why people feel both physically and emotionally exhausted after panicking.

Once, I was cooking pasta. I saw a huge moth. I panicked. I had to get out. I slammed the front door and went to my neighbours to ask them to get it. I locked us out and had to call a locksmith. The pan had gone dry. I worry I could have started a fire or something but I literally wasn't thinking straight. All I had on my mind was to escape.

Corinne

Frozen

We are all now acquainted with the term 'fight or flight', but we don't talk much about the 'freeze' state. It's a rare and often lifesaving response to trauma. The nervous system is overwhelmed so the usual coping mechanisms and responses are bypassed. The mind and body shut down in order to dissociate you from the trauma of the situation. It's not a conscious or rational process but something the body is wired to do.

In a split second the mind concludes that it will neither be able to fight or flee the threat. Therefore, the best and most protective state is to switch off entirely. The body is flooded with natural pain relief to numb any physical pain.

Consider how animals play dead when faced with direct attack. This isn't something they have chosen to do out of intelligent decision making, rather they have made a lightning speed, unconscious observation that they will neither survive the fight or flight. Sometimes this saves their life, as the 'shut down' can be so convincing.

I had a really difficult birth as there was an issue with the cord. There's a huge chunk of the labour that I literally cannot remember. My husband said I was suddenly rushed into theatre and it was scary, but all I remember is the midwife pushing the button and then suddenly hearing all these feet down the corridor. Then I remember nothing, even though my husband swears I was awake. I've had quite a bit of therapy since then, and my therapist said that it was my mind's way of blocking everything out to try and lessen the impact of the trauma on my mind.

Tia

Where am I on that line?

We move along that line constantly. We may have patches of time where we linger more towards one end than the other or bob around the centre. It's good to consider where you spend most of your time and how quickly it takes you to hop from one position to another.

Next time you have a strong feeling, observe where you might have moved along the line and what may have triggered that shift. Identify the feelings that have come with it, both physically and emotionally, and what it does to your energy levels too. This awareness can really help you as you learn more about yourself and what prompts you to be nudged or catapulted up or down the line.

I'm always a bit worried. Isn't that just part of the job description of being a mum? It comes with the territory.

Esther

Hearing the white noise

You may have 'generalised anxiety' or some other similar label in your doctor's notes. You may have self-diagnosed after reading about anxiety in books or online. Perhaps you recognise the general feeling of fear bubbling in the background like white noise that has become part of the soundtrack to your life.

Sometimes I realise how normal anxiety has become for me. It's like part of who I am and I have to remind myself about times that I've felt more relaxed so that I know that it can be better, and to encourage myself to address it.

Anonymous

I use white noise a lot for Florence's naps when out and about. I have a machine that plays noise in her buggy. I forget it's there. So many times I have walked into a shop and people have stopped to look round. Has someone left a tap running? Is there a gas leak? I spot their confused faces and explain.

The noise that my ears have blocked out is so loud to them. Sometimes I've forgotten to turn her white noise off because it has blended into the background. She may be happily awake before I realise that the sound is still blasting unnecessarily. I switch it off. Wow – the quiet that follows where before there had been a roar.

Anxiety doesn't have to be the background buzz.

We become so used to our own thought processes and anxieties. We can begin to accept them as 'part of who we are', or 'just the way I think'. Then, we forget how loud and impactful they are. We become almost immune to the bearing they have on our emotions and headspace.

We forget how it used to feel to have a more calm mind. Shoulders that felt less tense. Feet that meandered. A mind that could focus because it wasn't so scattered and worried.

Does anyone else feel a tad smug when someone tells you your shoulders are tense? I do! I don't know why a part of me wears tension like a badge of honour. I'm often battling with the part of my mind that tells me that if I'm not rushing, I'm not doing enough. If I'm not worrying, I'm not loving enough. If I'm not tense, I'm not carrying enough – mentally, emotionally, physically. If I'm not stretched to my max, I should be doing more. How unkind to put such pressure on ourselves. No wonder we feel anxious. It's like there's a mini-me standing over me waving a baton going, 'More. More.'

We get used to feeling anxious. It comes with the territory right? Whilst I would have agreed a few years ago, sighed and eye-rolled with a half-smile, it saddened me because I now believe there is more for all of us. I honestly believe that anxiety doesn't have to be the background buzz. Fear doesn't have to be such a factor in the decisions we make for our children and ourselves. It doesn't have to be the white noise we acclimatise to.

When I started addressing anxiety with my therapist, I suddenly realised how much of my days and my mood it had impacted.

Tamsin

In many ways, it's great that social media gets us talking openly about some of our feelings and thoughts as mothers. Laughing about mum guilt and the common anxieties. We feel less alone, but is that enough? Are we recognising that what we actually need to do is turn that annoying white noise down? It is possible to turn it down. I have. I do. You can. I know where the controls are now.

Anxiety – why it's helpful to know what's really going on

You know what anxiety feels like, now let's look at the whats and the whys, the hows and the whens.

The whats and the whys can really help you regain some control back from anxiety. I did antenatal classes. I went predominantly to make friends. I remember slowly studying the mums-to-be around me, how they seemed to be balancing on the edge of such life change. It was good. Strangers quickly became friends. And friends became allies as we navigated that first year of motherhood like drunken sailors on a swaying boat. Amidst the fake babies, swaddling techniques, breathing exercises and birthing positions, the most helpful thing for me was the knowledge of what happens to the body during labour.

We were educated on the nitty gritty of the hormones at play, what they did and how they worked. We were taught about the interplay between adrenaline, noradrenaline, oxytocin and endorphins. This was valuable because when labour came, whilst unknown and new, I had some idea of the process happening to me. It made it less scary, less unpredictable. I knew there was some sort of natural order to what was happening.

In moments of clarity, I recalled how using the breathing techniques would physiologically reduce the stress hormone cortisol, and make space for oxytocin, which helps labour progress. Knowledge meant that I didn't feel completely passive to the process of labour, I felt active within it. There were things I could do to help.

This is an example of how knowledge can help with excessive worry and anxiety. Know that it doesn't have to be this way. Know that it doesn't have to feel like you're a victim of your thoughts. Anxiety doesn't have to be at the helm of your ship on the stormy sea. *You* are at the helm.

Anxiety is the waves. They come and go, ebb and flow, but you are in control of the sails, the direction, the way the boat cuts through the chaos.

So, let's acquire some knowledge. I promise you it's not going to be a heavy science lesson. It's going to be help-ful. I'm going to help you see how you have more control over the mental and physical aspect of anxiety than you think you do.

Anxiety isn't all bad

Whilst anxiety may get a bad rap, it can be a good thing in its stripped-back form. We seem to recognise anxiety as a medical diagnosis typed into a doctor's records. It's a label we've adopted to describe something negative that needs to be fixed, or tiptoed around, or sympathised with. I remember being told as a young teen that our family friend was 'anxious'. I instantly had an image of a piece of fragile glass at risk of shattering and felt we'd better be gentle with her.

As a result, we often focus on the worst parts of anxiety. We only give it airtime when it feels overwhelming or you're sick of it and it needs to be addressed. But anxiety also serves as a protective mechanism, an energising life force to keep us safe. Without it, you wouldn't give safety a second thought because you wouldn't be considering risks or possibilities.

The word 'anxiety' makes me think of bad feelings.

Fran

Without anxiety, you wouldn't experience that energising rush of adrenaline you get before attempting a new task or challenge. Or the buzz of excitement when you anticipate something great happening.

Anxiety acts as your body's inbuilt warning system. It's a red light telling you that something is awry, in an attempt to draw your attention to it so that you can rectify the problem. The other day, we strolled along the Mumbles promenade in Wales. The boys ran up to the seafront railings and Charlie began to lean. The gaps between the railings were very wide, more than wide enough for him to flip through should he lean too far. On seeing this, I immediately felt anxiety. It was a rush of energy that came into my body and I envisioned him tumbling into the sea whilst pointing out a seagull.

Anxiety can be life-saving on occasions, and life-restricting in others.

With a burst of energy, my legs ran forward and I gently pulled them back from the railings. I told them they could look and point just as well from there. My brain processed that moment as a risk, prompting me to act, and giving me an injection of adrenaline-fuelled energy to do so.

The body processes fear and excitement in the same way, which is why you might notice that physically, they echo each other. What makes the difference between whether we perceive something as a good or bad feeling is the way our brain interprets the thing that triggers our anxiety response.

The caveman

This might sound strange, but I want you to imagine a caveman. A tall, sturdy, hairy chap with the kind of muscle you can't sculpt at the gym. He's built from spending his days gathering, hunting, carrying, climbing, striding. He comes back to his cave and throws down the spoils of his hunting. The fire is full and the flames are hungrily licking the simmering dinner pot above them. Suddenly, the threatening roar of a bear enters the cave and ricochets off the walls.

In milliseconds, the caveman's senses have sent lightning-speed signals to the amygdala area in his brain, which is responsible for processing and responding to emotion. A sudden electrical storm of activity assesses the roar and interprets it as a threat to his family, his life and his safety. This information signals the hypothalamus in the brain to immediately prepare his body to either fight the bear or gather his family and run for their lives.

Whether he chooses to fight or flee, both actions require an immense amount of effort from the nervous system. The nervous system is like the body's electrical wiring. Imagine bundles of sparking fibre cable that are at their most dense at the brain and spinal cord and then span out to every area of the body. It collects sensory input, processes it and tells the body how to respond.

Suddenly the adrenal glands pump out adrenaline (think downing a line-up of espressos), both breathing and heart rates increase and eyes dilate to see better. Our caveman is alert, on edge, ready and raring to fight or run. The stress hormone cortisol then gets pumped into the blood stream to help the body sustain this response.

As the roar of the bear passes and the threat lessens, the cortisol and the adrenaline slowly diminish, leaving the caveman to return to a more relaxed state. It's mealtime and he can relax and focus on eating now he's not at risk of being the meal.

The day my mother-in-law's nervous system saved my life!

These fight or flight reactions can undoubtedly save your life at the times you need it. It can give people seemingly superhuman strength and speed that do not occur in day-to-day life. You hear of people finding strength to lift a car. I'll never forget the moment in which my mother-in-law literally saved my life.

We were crossing a busy road and I lifted my foot to step out at a central island, expecting traffic on the single lane road to come from my left. An arm flew across my body, sharply pushing me back onto the pavement. As it happened, a bus flew mere centimetres past my face from my right. Within milliseconds, her nervous system saw a threat, assessed the risk and told her arm to save me. It took us a while to process what had happened and for our hearts to slow down.

Devastatingly, my husband's good friend had been killed merely weeks before at that same crossing where traffic wasn't directed in a way that was expected by pedestrians. The whole area has since been reconfigured. In that moment, my mother-in-law's fight or flight response saved my life. But coincidentally it also worked to fuel my anxiety, as I was so struck by what could have been and reminded of the fragility of life. I endured flashbacks for a while as I processed it.

However, these moments of real physical threat are few and far between. That lifesaving nervous system response isn't often required.

The impact of anxiety when our lives are safe

But what happens when we experience anxious thoughts when we aren't physically threatened? We hold on to these anxious or intrusive thoughts and we make them big with our creative minds. They snowball into threats that feel real and possible and huge and scary, and then that 'caveman' nervous system response is triggered.

We don't need to fight or flee, but our mind tells our body that our lives, safety and peace are in dire jeopardy.

When I start to worry about something happening to Chelle, I can feel my whole body rev up like an engine. You know, when you press on the accelerator of a car really hard but it's not in gear? It's like that.

Hazel

Life is risky. Many of us are more aware of our own vulnerability than we would like to be. All living organisms are vulnerable to things inside and outside of our control. It's a permanent state of being alive. My parents protected us from many things within their control. We wore seatbelts, ate a fairly balanced diet. We learnt to cross roads safely and not insert forks into plug sockets. But they could not protect my sister from the cancer that grew of its own accord within her brain.

There are moments in life where that reality comes into painfully sharp focus and it can feel overwhelming and scary. But, there's so much hope. A lot of addressing anxiety is about finding ways to anchor yourself amidst the fragility of life. It's about coming to terms with all the coulds and the mights and finding joy and peace amidst them, not in spite of them. I promise you that is possible. I really do.

Anxiety isn't all bad in itself. It's actually valuable. However, you're here because you want more. You want to believe there's more to motherhood than the frantic late-night internet searches, the ever-present fear that something is going to happen to your baby, or the ability to cry at the drop of a coin. I wanted more too. And there is more and it makes all the difference.

Sometimes I feel like there must be another way to think. My awareness of what could go wrong is like a shadow over the nice times.

Inca

I'll give you an example of when anxiety robs me in the small moments. I remember snuggling seven-month-old Florence into my chest. I Inhaled her. I revelled in that feeling for a second. I drank it in. Then BAM. It was suddenly interrupted by an intrusive anxious thought. What if she died? What if something bad were to happen? What if she got sick? Quickly that sumptuous mindful moment of love became fear-based. Instead of holding her close out of enjoyment, I held her close out of fear. Joy became fear. Anxiety turns peace, calm, mindfulness and joy . . . into fear and trepidation.

A while ago, that fear would have swallowed me up and sat like a dead weight in the pit of my stomach, stirring up that fight or flight response, causing me to act, to retreat, to be hypersensitive to risk. Yet these days, I let it move on by. I did some long exhales to tell my nervous system to calm. There's no immediate threat. Then I grounded myself, imagining the most statistically likely scenario of her visiting me in my old age, as a grandmother rocking in a well-loved chair. (That worked for me, but I'll give you many tips and techniques to try if this isn't your bag.)

See, I'm not immune to anxious thoughts. None of us are. But they have significantly less impact on my actions, my feelings and my sense of self than they did. And that *is* attainable. It's liberating when you realise you don't have to be at their mercy.

Top tip

When you feel anxious, breathe in through your nose to the count of four and out through your mouth to the count of six.

JOURNAL POINTS

- Where on the line do you spend most of your time? Has it always been this way?
- Recall the last time you felt content and relaxed. What enabled you to feel that way?
- Consider the things that trigger your anxiety. Are they internal or external?
- Have you ever experienced anxiety in a positive way?

Chapter 3

The many masks of anxiety

Mantra: *Anxiety can't thrive when we focus on the present.*

Anxiety is like a very refined con artist, a master of disguise. Strip away the cloak and stick-on moustache and it comes down to the same three things:

1.   Fear of bad things happening
2.   A need to feel in control
3.   Not feeling good enough

Anxiety likes a focus point, it likes to ruminate, obsess and fixate. But it can also change shape. By getting to know its various guises, we can start to see where it is at work in our lives. I'm going to take you through many of the masks of anxiety, starting with the ways in which it has manifested in my own life along the years.

The various masks of my anxiety

In the past, my anxiety has presented itself in many different ways. It feels quite a vulnerable thing to let you in on this, because often we feel ashamed of these behaviours and prefer to keep them secret, out of fear of judgement or being thought of as 'mad'. But as I'm encouraging you to consider the ways your anxiety has manifested over the years and some of the guises it has held, it seems only fair that I lead by example.

Whilst anxiety might make you feel ashamed, that shame isn't justified.

Also, I want to show you that whilst anxiety might make you feel ashamed, that shame isn't justified. Shame keeps us stuck and feeling alone in the buzzing world inside our minds. The most effective way to dismantle this undeserving shame is to talk about the very things we are ashamed of. So, here goes.

I first experienced anxiety as a child when my sister was diagnosed with a brain tumour. After her diagnosis, I would feel constant fear that someone else in my life would get sick. The prognosis of her cancer was that she would hopefully enter a period of remission, but ultimately the cancer would be terminal. When discovered, it was the size of a man's fist.

When they operated on her, they were forced to leave a sliver of tumour, the size of a 50p piece (back then, 50p coins were larger than the dainty ones we have now). I was ten when she died. I remember being preoccupied with all the things that could go wrong should a family member leave my immediate vicinity. My anxiety could only be reassured by their return.

I would join my brother on playdates with his friends, claiming I wanted to go, but in truth the drive was fear that something would happen. This fear felt intolerable when I thought about it for more than a second. It would make me feel sick. I used to tell myself that it was OK, because if anyone else died, I would ensure I died too in order to escape the pain of another loss.

The next manifestation of my anxiety that I remember was an intense and terrifying fear of vomiting. So intense was this fear that I ran across a busy road once without checking for traffic in order to escape someone vomiting. I wasn't sick for an entire decade, as my body simply wouldn't lean into illness in that way.

Everywhere I went, I'd be scanning the ground and people's faces, looking for risk. If someone coughed a certain way, or gagged, I'd panic and bolt. I'd avoid certain events and places where people were more likely to be sick. Aeroplanes and travel put me on high alert. I had various forms of therapy over the years in order to address this. Hyperemesis (all day, acute sickness) in two of my pregnancies made sure that my own sickness is less of an anxiety trigger for me now. Now, the sickness, or threatened sickness, of others still spikes my anxiety and triggers the fight or flight response but I no longer live in daily fear as I now have solid coping mechanisms to help me.

I've also experienced an obsessive-compulsive manifestation of anxiety. For a long period of time I was obsessed with counting. I'd count calories. I'd count steps walked and climbed. My head would be constantly filled with numbers. I'd know how many steps it took to get me from one room to another, from my office to the shop. I'd know the number of stairs in the places I frequented and would feel a compulsive need to count them regardless of knowing there were two sets of twelve per floor. This compulsion ensured that numbers filled every nook of my mind like roaring noise that drowned out other feelings and anxieties. It gave me a strange sense of control and ownership, but at the same time I felt at the mercy of it. I couldn't seem to stop.

At other times in my life, during transitions of sorts, such as a house move or my first weeks at university, I've clung to physical order. In my university accommodation, I had a room to myself. Life felt new and exciting, chaotic and adventurous. My room became my haven. If life lacked order, my room would make up for it. Everything had its place and whilst I loved hosting pre-party drinks and movie nights, I felt a constant fizz of anxiety at things being nudged and moved, picked up and shuffled. Once everyone left I'd feel relief as I tweaked positions and replaced things where they belonged. Order was restored, physically and mentally.

Driving is another area my anxiety likes to focus on. Driving anxiety is very common, whereby people find it hard to overlook the risks associated with driving. It can range in severity from being hesitant to drive to refusing to do so at all. I won't go into too much depth here but the most prominent part of my driving anxiety was the intrusive thoughts I would have about crashing my car or being in a pile-up.

I very clearly remember the first time it totally floored

me that intrusive thoughts were a 'thing' and not the result of my brain being broken. I was at a family gathering celebrating my relatives' wedding anniversary. My brother and I were standing against a fence in a sunny pub garden. He had a bottle of beer in his hand, I had a glass of wine. He turned to me and said, 'Do you ever get funny thoughts, like, I could break this bottle against the fence and run into the crowd? Obviously, I'd never do it but do you ever get thoughts like that?'

It was one of the most memorable moments of my mental health journey. Suddenly, something I'd shrouded with so much shame and secrecy was being spoken about. I could absolutely identify. From thoughts of pushing over a loaded display stand of mugs in cluttered gift shops, to swiftly pulling a stranger's ponytail. And darker thoughts like jumping off Waterloo Bridge into the icy Thames as I walked to work, or deftly turning my wheel on the motorway and causing a tragic pile-up.

I didn't know what these strange thoughts were but for the first time in my life, I knew I wasn't alone in having them. Immense relief followed. Chapter 8 focuses on the dynamics of intrusive thoughts – the knowledge and insight on how to deal with them have been life-changing for me, and I hope it may help you too.

What about now?

I still get a mixture of all of these manifestations of anxiety to varying degrees. Anxiety loves a focus. It's hugely dependent on what's going on in my life and mind, whether I've been investing time and space to care for my wellbeing or not. It depends on stress levels and hormones, and how much sleep I've had.

I can confidently tell you that none of these things impact my daily life in the way they used to. They rarely rob me of enjoyment; they have little to no impact in the decisions I make for me and my children. I don't avoid events or experiences anymore. As I type, seven-month-old Florence has been kindly taken out of the house for an hour so that I can focus on these words. Fleeting thoughts were, *something's going to happen to her whilst out of my care. I'll never see her again. What if she chokes on her snack?* Years ago, I would have wanted her to stay here, driven by those fears. But I'm glad I can now see them for what they are, and that she can go out, see the ducks, get some fresh air and some undivided attention.

Recently I'd heard of a stomach bug circling Charlie's nursery like a hungry shark. As soon as I was told by one of the practitioners when I arrived to drop him off, my immediate desire was to bundle him back into the car and keep him home for the rest of the week. But I saw the anxious thoughts and the swelling feeling of panic for what they were. I breathed the fear away and watched him run off to find his friends. If I had leaned into my fear, I may have slightly lessened his risk of sickness but I'd have certainly lessened his chance of fun and adventure with his friends.

My anxiety has many guises but ultimately the same essence in each – a sense of lack of control and a fear of bad things happening. I hope that gives you insight into some of the various ways anxiety can manifest. Anxiety can be like that whack-a-mole game at the fair. You whack one of the plastic moles on its head with the mallet and another one immediately pops up somewhere else.

Addressing the symptoms and the causes

Many approaches to treating anxiety address the symptoms fabulously but neglect the cause. Unless we address the cause and the common veins that run deeply through all these different manifestations, binding them together, we will see it pop up in another form later on. A multi-pronged attack is always beneficial, which is why I advocate therapy alongside the tips and tools I share.

Many approaches for treating anxiety address the symptoms fabulously but neglect the cause.

Anxiety switches off the rational, problem-solving and calmer part of the brain. I'm going to help equip you with the insight and tools to help switch it back on so you can start claiming control back from anxiety's clutches.

Anxiety switches off the rational, problem-solving and calmer part of the brain.

What can anxiety feel like?

Before looking at common focuses of anxiety, have a glance over this list of physical and mental symptoms. This ensures that we're all singing from the same hymn sheet when we talk about anxiety. But it could also be helpful for you to identify which ones you experience and any symptoms you might have not linked to anxiety before.

Physical symptoms

- Panic attacks
- Nausea
- Tension in the body, e.g. sore back or shoulders, headaches
- Clenching jaw and maybe grinding teeth
- Fast or inconsistent heart rate
- Problems falling and staying asleep
- Hot flushes or sweating
- Restlessness
- Light-headedness and/or increased breathing rate
- Churning stomach or loose bowel movements
- Pins and needles
- Dips in energy and/or sex drive

Mental symptoms

- Feeling dissociated (disconnected) from your mind, body, the world or reality.
- Craving reassurance from others

- Being unable to relax
- Struggling to control worries
- Increased sensitivity to what others say or do, or what they might think about you
- Ruminating (thinking over and over something)
- Worrying about the future
- Fearing panic attacks
- Feeling like everything around you is going very quickly or slowly

Common focuses of anxiety

Here are some common forms of anxiety. Have a read and see if you relate to any of them.

General anxiety

Generalised anxiety can be described as a feeling of anxiety and tension without knowing the specific cause or trigger. Generalised anxiety is different for everyone: some may experience more physical symptoms, like a fast heart rate and a stomach that feels like a washing machine, while others may experience more mental symptoms, like tornadoes of spiralling thoughts that are hard to stop. Anxiety impacts the mind and body in many different ways, so one person's experience may look totally different to another's.

I honestly don't know where the feelings come from. I can be going about my day and start to feel like everything is moving fast and then my breathing goes funny and I start thinking something bad is going to happen. It might be a thought I have and don't realise that kicks it off. I have to sit down and breathe and try to get a handle on stuff.

Anonymous

Obsessive-compulsive disorder (OCD)

OCD is a strong compulsion to use specific rituals to control anxious thoughts, in an attempt to stop things from happening. These behaviours tend to fall into the following categories: fear of contamination, ordering objects in particular ways, thoughts of harming others, compulsive checking or repeated aggressive, sexual thoughts.

I read about a ten-month-old kid dying from complications of food poisoning from bad chicken. I got totally obsessed and scared. I wouldn't feed Cam any meat. I told everyone he was allergic to meat. It felt like it would certainly happen if he ate meat. I made our household into a vegetarian one and got very anxious if he ate away from home.

Janelle

These behaviours are likely to have emerged at a time when the individual felt unsafe. Repeated behaviours can initially offer a much-yearned for sense of control. It's not a personality trait despite the fact it has wrongly become a colloquial phrase, *Oh, I'm so OCD*, adopted by those who are describing rigidity or a strong desire for order or cleanliness. It's a psychological disorder that has come about in a desperate grapple for control but, ironically, the compulsion ends up holding all the keys. Obsessions and actions become so addictive and compulsive that they impact daily life and trigger huge anxiety if they cannot be fulfilled.

> *I missed the flight to my sister's wedding because I had to continually return home to check the gas hob wasn't on. It was then I realised how much these compulsions were stealing from me. I saw a therapist the next week.*
>
> Emma

If these words really resonate for you right now, even in a small way, I promise there's hope. This book will go some way to help address the anxiety you feel but ultimately therapy plays the most valuable and important part in reclaiming back your life and your headspace. If at any point you feel you'd benefit, please seek additional support. Your GP is a great first point of contact and will be able to advise you further.

> *I became absolutely obsessed with sudden infant death syndrome (SIDS). For three months I would wake up every twenty or so minutes to check on my baby. I'd search on the internet for hours each day for tips on how to avoid it. I spent a lot of money on gadgets and sensor mats, and 'stuff'. I bumped my car because I was so tired. My friends intervened and I got help. I hadn't realised how bad it got but they could see. Things have settled down now I have addressed something that happened in my family that I'd swept under the carpet. I still get OCD-type things but I've got some good help and tricks up my sleeve to help.*
>
> Addy

Compulsive behaviour

Closely linked to OCD, compulsive behaviour is often self-destructive and habitual behaviour that is driven by the need to ease internal feelings. Examples include skin picking, hair pulling and dysfunctional relationships with food. Hoarding, shopping, gambling, checking and cleaning are further examples. It might be something done mindlessly, without realising, but the likelihood is that it's very regular and repetitive and ultimately feels hard to control.

> *I pick the skin on my lips. It's weird because I suddenly realise I'm doing it. Often, they look dry and will bleed. I feel like I should stop but it's hard to stop something you don't always know you're doing. I definitely do it more when I'm stressed or concentrating on something. Sometimes I really want to do it because there's a dry bit and I feel like I have to pick it off. I don't like talking about it and I feel like everyone is looking at my lips wondering if I'm allergic to something. I even sit on my hands sometimes.*
>
> Anonymous

It's not particularly rewarding. It might make the individual feel better in some small way as they act on the compulsion, like a burst of relief. But ultimately these behaviours can be harmful to varying degrees.

Post-traumatic stress disorder (PTSD)

PTSD is a very present fear resulting from something that happened involving physical or emotional harm or threat.

The trigger may be a single event such as a car crash or a traumatic birth. However, it can also be triggered by chronic, ongoing situations such as an emotionally abusive relationship or sexual abuse.

Here is a list of symptoms for you to look out for. It's not exhaustive or intended for self-diagnosis. It's a reference point for you. If you feel you might have PTSD to any degree, please speak with your GP or seek a therapist. You deserve to have space to address and process what you've been through in a gentle and supported way.

Symptoms may be:

- Emotional numbness
- Avoidance of anything that may act as a reminder
- Mental and/or physical response to reminders
- Trouble remembering all of the details of the event or events
- Decreased interest in the things usually enjoyed
- Feelings of detachment or desire to detach from others
- Difficulty sleeping or concentrating
- General irritation or anger
- Feeling low or depressed
- Re-experiencing the trauma through flashbacks or nightmares
- Feeling fearful and unsafe, and/or being hyper-vigilant
- Destructive behaviour

My baby had an undiagnosed bowel problem. All she did was scream. I'm not exaggerating. I couldn't leave the house. I started drinking wine at night to blot out the fact that I felt so helpless. I couldn't see a way through. Then my drinking increased and started earlier and earlier. I felt so ashamed but I didn't know what else to do. My husband and health visitor got me help and finally my baby got diagnosed. I quit drinking but I still get flashbacks and feel panicked when she cries because it takes me right back.

Anonymous

Not everyone who experiences a traumatic incident will go on to get PTSD. It's dependent on a large number of factors such as support network, resilience, historical experience, personality type and age. Also, what else is going on in life for the individual at that time, what other stressors are at play and the speed of support. If you experience PTSD, it's certainly not because you are weak or at fault.

Health anxiety

Health anxiety is common and can step up a gear in motherhood. Suddenly one feels all this love for a tiny being and it becomes inconceivable to lose them. Health anxiety is a preoccupation with the idea or fear that the individual themself is unwell or someone they care about. They might find themselves frequently checking for any signs or symptoms of illness and feel compelled to research them. Anxiety may be particularly triggered by hearing concerning stories about other people or their children becoming unwell. A rash or a temperature might initiate a spiral of fear and overthinking.

Decisions may be made based on fears, such as avoiding

playdates because one child has been unwell, or seeking advice and appointments for reassurance.

My friend's little boy was born with his bowel on the outside of his tummy. He had to have surgery and I saw how scary it was for them. So, when I was pregnant with Oliver, I spent hours on the internet researching the issue and the likelihood that my baby would have it too. I couldn't stop thinking about it. At times I felt almost certain that he had it too. Every time I had a scan, I would ask the sonographer to check and check again that his bowels were in the right place.

Marnie

Phobia

Phobias are an intense fear of a specific thing or situation. The sense of danger and fear the person experiences towards the object or situation is exaggerated and often triggers physical symptoms of panic. Individuals feel anxious when faced with the source of their phobia but even thinking about it may trigger panic in some.

Depending on the level, source and cause of the phobia, it can impact the sufferer's life to different degrees. One person may panic when exposed to a spider, whereas someone fearful of open spaces might avoid leaving the house because of it.

If you are struggling, I promise that your phobia does not need to forever impact your enjoyment of certain situations in the way it has done. There are many tips and tools in this book that will help you cope the next time you are faced with your trigger. But it's also beneficial to seek insight into when the phobia developed. It might be that you had a difficult experience that you need the opportunity to process, to help disempower the phobia.

> *I struggled with phobia of birth – tokophobia. It was so bad that I considered not having a baby at all. It was a surprise when I found out I was pregnant and my fear of labour consumed my whole pregnancy. I couldn't watch anything where someone gave birth or even talked about it because I'd start to panic. I didn't do any antenatal classes. My consultant agreed that I could have a planned c-section. I also had CBT and found a doula who really helped prepare me for the birth. It all went much better than I expected. We'd love another baby, so I'm going to have some counselling before we try to conceive because I don't want the phobia to ruin my enjoyment of another pregnancy.*

Anonymous

Social anxiety

Social anxiety is a form of phobia that impacts daily life. Someone who experiences social anxiety will feel anxious before social activities or may avoid certain activities altogether. When around others, they might feel very self-conscious, like they are being watched. Another symptom is to feel hyper-sensitive to the actions and responses of others, worrying that others are judging them or thinking negatively about them. After socialising, they may then find it hard to stop overthinking about the interactions they had.

Social anxiety can impact relationships and the enjoyment of life itself, as it is tricky to constantly avoid triggering situations. It is completely worth addressing, as it can make the world feel small and lonely. We are all worthy of enjoyable social interactions with one another.

I would literally sweat and shake before I walked into a room of people I didn't know. It felt like everyone was looking at me. When I left, I'd end up going through everything I said and did to make sure I hadn't embarrassed myself. I find it much easier now but sometimes I do get a wave of it and want to run away from social situations! I breathe through it and it does pass.

Siobhan

Panic disorder

Panic disorder is characterised by sudden panic attacks that seem to come out of the blue. A sufferer can become fearful of the panic attacks themselves, causing them to avoid situations that may trigger them. Panic disorder can become debilitating and impact the sufferer's quality of life.

If you have been experiencing regular panic attacks, I encourage you to speak with your GP or a therapist. With the correct support they can be addressed, often with great success!

I had a stressful situation with a boss at work. Suddenly I began having these panic attacks. At first, I honestly thought I was going to die. I felt like I couldn't breathe. My friend called an ambulance. Fortunately, my work restructured and stuff calmed down. I have tools to deal with the attacks when they happen, but it's quite rare now. I definitely think mine are linked to stress.

Anonymous

The anxiety rollercoaster

My husband works in London and often returns home after I'm in bed. There have been times when I've lain awake with horrendous, intrusive scenarios playing through my mind like elaborate theatre productions. I imagine him getting killed in a terrorist attack on the tube, me wracked with grief, wondering how to break it to the children. Then I begin to work out how I'd pay our mortgage alone and whether I'd go back to full-time work or have to move in with my parents. Before I know it, even though this is entirely made up, my heart has experienced stabs of grief, confusion and fear.

If only we were anxious about unlikely events: alien invasions, bears lurking under the bed ... it would be much easier to seek the reassurance and statistics needed to calm our anxious minds. You see, our anxieties contain some element of real-life possibility. We yearn for reassurance, but for anyone to promise us, hand on heart, that these fears would never come to fruition would be dishonest.

Anxiety can cause you to experience a rollercoaster of very real emotion irrespective of whether you're lying in a dark room or sitting on a train. You can be whizzing through fearful scenarios in your mind's eye and nobody would notice. Anxiety causes your mind to race ahead at 100mph, from where things are (probably) OK into a fabricated future where they are definitely not.

All anxiety ends up doing is causing you emotional distress in the present, sucking away the contentment you could be experiencing. You cannot be anxious and present at the same time. An anxious mind cannot be running ahead into an unknown future whilst being fully present in what you're doing. We are going to find ways to help you be more present in the moment, so that anxiety can't thrive.

> **You cannot be anxious and present at the same time.**

Top Tip

Familiarise yourself with the different symptoms of anxiety and start to observe which of them are relevant to you and when they pop up. Make a short note of the trigger and symptom.

JOURNAL POINTS

- What does anxiety feel like to you?
- What are the different ways in which your anxiety has manifested?
- Did anything in this chapter particularly jump out at you?

▶

- Is there any area in which you'd benefit from some additional insight or support? How might you access that?
- Anxiety often comes down to three things (see page 41) – which category or categories do most of your anxious thoughts sit in?

Chapter 4

Are we living in anxious times?

Mantra: *Calm is the balm we need.*

I often get asked, 'Are we more anxious than generations before us? Or is it that we're more aware of what anxiety is?' Were previous generations as impacted by the sense of lack of control and worry that we seem to be so accepting of these days?

I recently discussed this with my mum (a fellow therapist) one evening. She offered such brilliant insight I thought I'd share it with you. I'm going to list many recent cultural shifts that fuel the maternal anxiety that seems to shape so much of our parenting experience. I've also peppered it with responses to the question I put to my social media following: Are we a more anxious generation? If so, why?'

Emotional management

Then

It seems apt to start by questioning whether there has been a shift in how we manage emotions. I remember my grandfather used to say, 'don't cry' whenever we burst into tears. He was loving and firm, but, for him, difficult emotions were private and to be replaced with a positive mental attitude. Our parents were likely raised by the war-touched 'keep calm, carry on' generation. Bravery was praised, so fears and anxiety were pushed down.

It may also be that anxiety was more stigmatised and less understood and anyone who was anxious may have been labelled 'a bit neurotic' or 'a worrier'. Anxiety and other mental health challenges were perhaps viewed as character flaws, rather than cycles of thoughts that one could actually address and free yourself from.

I do wonder whether older generations, who lived in just as disruptive political and economic times, were simply forced to bottle it all up. A relative's first-born baby died during labour in the 1950s. She never spoke of it again but every time a baby was born she would be on edge until she had heard all was well. Looking back on how she dealt with various things, especially health, this was anxiety but she was labelled 'a worrier' by everyone.

Anonymous

Now

I used to believe that my sometimes relentless worried and anxious thoughts were 'just the way I was wired'. I didn't realise that I could equip my mind with tools and techniques to challenge them.

My first experience of therapy was when my parents realised I had a phobia of vomiting (called emetophobia – it's surprisingly common). It was potentially tied to the traumatic symptoms of my sister's cancer but, from the age of ten, this fear started to dictate the choices I made; it impacted my ability to enjoy social occasions and I became increasingly fearful of encountering sickness on a day-to-day basis.

I went for some therapy with a kindly lady who taught me that with a bit of work, there was hope. And there was hope. It no longer rules my life. And there is hope for you, regardless of what challenge you face or secret fear you hold.

Now, thanks to the internet, more research, funding and awareness, we are increasingly understanding that anxiety is something we can address should we want to. It doesn't have to be 'how we are'; it doesn't have to impact our daily choices and behaviour.

There are constant campaigns aimed at de-stigmatising mental health conditions. Those in the media spotlight are choosing to speak out about things that would have once been shut away like shameful secrets. Conversations are being started, resources being made increasingly available. We're not there yet but we're certainly making inroads.

We are better at talking about it now. Even eight or so years ago when I was first diagnosed with anxiety, it wasn't something people talked about. Now I am very open about it.

Nathalie

Headspace

Then

A generation ago, work stopped and then home life began. If you were lucky, you had four exciting TV channels to skip through to give you some escapism. A small collection of videos sat on a shelf (often carefully recorded, and we'd be in trouble if we put one back in its cardboard case without re-winding it), and kids' TV was bookended at sociable hours by the static picture of a smiling clown, telling you that it was too late or too early for TV.

Favourite programmes would be circled on weekly magazines in biro and adverts would act as tea or loo breaks. You had to watch, otherwise you'd miss out on a twist or the opportunity for a laugh. Perhaps you'd read a good book, its corner turned down waiting for you to resume. There were board games and phone calls that you'd pick up not knowing who was on the end of the line. Computers? What are they? Wi-Fi? What is this language you speak of?

Toys, there weren't tonnes of them, they weren't cheap. We had secondhand toys bought from toy sales or passed on by friends. Play was lower sensory, rarely did anything flash and sing, whirr or beep. As kids we'd spend hours role-playing, hiding, dressing up and re-enacting memories and things we'd seen.

Our favourite game used to be to dress up in my mum's old wedding dress and perform wedding ceremonies with each other, or to create makeshift spacecrafts, dressed in my metallic gymnastic leotards as the characters we glimpsed in my dad's fuzzily recorded sci-fi shows.

Now

Expectations are through the roof. The pressure (self-imposed or otherwise) is suffocating; plodding along at your own pace is no longer OK. Juggling hundreds of balls at once, though, now that will get you to the top of the league table, with a fast-track pass to burnout.

Liv

Life doesn't pause. It simply doesn't stop. You can switch on your TV to one of hundreds of channels at any time of the day or night. We often spend so long looking for the perfect film on a weekend night that by the time we've finally chosen one, I'm too tired to watch the whole thing before retreating blurry eyed to bed.

You can constantly refresh your social media feeds at 3 a.m. for an update of images and information to ping instantly to the bright screen in your hand. Emails, messages, texts, new podcasts . . . anything can come at any time.

There is hardly any stopping. Work merges into home life and then the boundaries between work and rest begin to blur. Nothing really begins and ends unless you consciously switch off and shut out the outside world but, even then, your inside world buzzes like static because you know that communication and all the calls for your attention are building up, waiting for you to switch back on and plug back in.

> We don't switch off and let our brains process healthily in the same way.
>
> Blum

Hours are long and the juggle is intense. So many times, colleagues of mine have scrambled out of meetings. They'd stuff papers into bags whilst muttering something about their partner forgetting it was their day for nursery pickup.

> We're a sandwich generation. We want to be our mothers but love our job.
>
> Marisa

Life is more expensive: commuting, childcare, borrowing money for mortgages. As a result, we wear so many different hats and find ourselves switching them constantly. We are sold the belief that we can do it all, yet the reality is that we feel like we're running on a treadmill with the speed set too high for our legs.

Instead of being able to compartmentalise life into filling wedges of cake, we

We are sold the belief that we can do it all yet the reality is that we feel like we're running on a treadmill with the speed set too high for our legs.

are forced to whittle them down into unappetising slivers that leave us hungry and unsatisfied. I often feel like everyone and everything gets a tiny piece of me, yet I'm longing for more compartmentalisation.

I'd love more quality time with the kids, away from the demands of the house, of life, of the technology relentlessly pinging for my attention. Time to do the work without my attention being dragged in thirty different directions. I'd like time with my husband without only being able to grunt simple logistics at the end of long days because we're both worn out in entirely different ways. Doing everything but feeling like I'm always failing slightly because there's not enough of me to go around.

Does that sound familiar? When did we start feeling like our own resources quite simply weren't enough, because the demands placed upon us (by ourselves or by culture ... or both) are simply too much for one human to fully attend to.

Toys bleep, flash and sing. I have the electronic tunes of Florence's bouncer on loop in my head as I try to sleep. We recently halved the number of toys in my kids' playroom, as their idea of play was to get them all out. They haven't even noticed.

We're bombarded. Noise, activity, connection all the time. Space isn't enforced by lack of anything. We're switched on more than ever and we're tired and stressed. Our consistent high-alert, switched-on state means that cortisol (stress) levels are higher, and as a result, we feel buzzing.

> **Our lifestyles are giving our bodies the signal that we are under stress and at risk.**

Our lifestyles are giving our bodies the signal that we are under stress and at risk, triggering our fight or flight mode. This prevents us finding the calm that is the balm we need.

Advice and information

Then

Needed information? The only options were chatting on the phone (which cost a pretty penny) to a friend or family member who'd 'been there, done that' and could hopefully impart some wisdom born from their own experience. Or asking a friend as you bumped into them at a playgroup, or as you ran an errand in town.

Alternatively, if it was a medical question you could book an appointment to talk to someone who was more likely to know the answer than you were, due to professional insight.

Or, you'd wing it, guided by your intuition. If it felt right, looked right, and your kid was OK, then it probably was right. And if it wasn't . . . you'll do something different next time. As long as the kids were safe and happy, it didn't really matter.

Now

Our intuition is so often drowned out by the buzz of every other accessible opinion. We believe there's an answer to everything somewhere if you look hard enough. Although, the more you look, the more confusing it is to uncover what the *right* answer *actually* is. As we are in constant pursuit of answers, we're losing touch with the still, small, quiet voice that *feels* right, regardless of what the noise around us says.

We fail to trust our gut instincts anymore.

Paz

I remember when, at four months old, Oscar seemed really unwell. We'd spent time at a friend's house. Everyone had concluded that he was teething. Out came the teething salts, and the sticky syringes, yet the screaming didn't abate.

Early the next morning, I stirred from an incredibly unsettled night with an undeniable feeling that something was very wrong. It felt like my stomach was weighted with jagged-edged boulders, yet my chest was bursting with a thousand restless butterflies. I called an ambulance and Oscar later had emergency bowel surgery. I won't go into the details of the whats and the whys, because, if you're anything like me, you'll add the entire scenario to your internal filing cabinet of 'all the bad things that *could potentially* happen'.

Anyway, the moral of my story was that amidst the tug of war of other people's subjective opinions on every single facet of parenting and motherhood, there's *your* opinion, *your* sense, *your* maternal intuition.

The more conflicting opinions we are exposed to, the more we are likely to second guess ourselves. This provokes anxiety due to fear of getting it wrong. And whilst it may well be important to seek the opinions of friends, family and professionals, listen to your gut too.

We have more info. So instead of fleeting thoughts we can over analyse now.

Viktoria

Bad and sad stories

Then

In our parents' generation, you'd catch the news at specific times of the day, perhaps on TV or you'd grab a newspaper. Stories closer to home would come through the grapevine of gossip and overheard conversation. Occasionally we'd catch wind of a tragic accident, a stillbirth, a car crash or a cancer diagnosis, and you'd be filled with concern and compassion for the families affected.

Bad and tragic things didn't happen every day to everyone, they weren't common occurrences. They didn't feel like it either. You didn't know all the possible illnesses and dangerous scenarios the world had to offer, because, unless they were newsworthy, or happened to a friend of a friend of a friend, you'd never have heard of them.

Now

These days, tragic and sad stories feel like everyday occurrences, everyday realities that could happen to us. Within our hands and on our screens, we are connected to hundreds of thousands of stories per day, not just the ones heard about on the 10 p.m. news or because your mum spent the evening on the phone to your aunt.

You'll find a pocket of community online for every single life experience and eventuality, which is amazing when it comes to being hungry for support from those who know what you're going through. But, find yourself down a social media rabbit-hole of mothers who have experienced loss when hunting for SIDS prevention tips, and suddenly the risk feels like it's gone from a tragic rarity to an almost certainty.

There are such wider reporting and awareness of dangers in the world.
Di

I remember the day that I watched a documentary and learnt about an obscure and rare cause of death I'd never heard of before. I'd never heard of it because it has never affected anyone I know. However, I got 'the fear' and headed to the internet to arm myself with knowledge of all potential symptoms should someone I know be afflicted. Because then I'd know, right? I could tell that person, save their life. Steer a tragedy from our paths.

As I skim-read the reams of digital information in my hands, I fell upon so many news articles, forums, stories and first-hand experiences that, in my mind, it rapidly got promoted from 'so rare that I'd never heard of it', to a very real threat that would most likely affect my family at some point.

The sheer volume of information we consume, that we

gulp down unknowingly during mindless scrolls, and that we seek out, hungry to get the information we so hope will calm our minds, contorts our reality. It distorts statistical likelihoods and ratios, like a wonky circus mirror that warps reality into something our brains struggle to process.

We feel hungry for information because we believe it will ground us. But too much, from too many sources, is more likely to give us the stability of a vulnerable boat in a raging ocean. No wonder we're all a bit anxious. The more we know about the risks, challenges and potentials of life, the more vulnerable we feel to the possibilities.

Friendships

Then

We grew up in a small village in Herefordshire. We knew neighbours, we had friends we saw regularly. We'd never get further than the veg shop before bumping into someone we knew. We'd hang off mum's leg as she chatted to her friends about boring grown-up things.

The longest journey we'd regularly make was on a Sunday where we'd do the 50-minute trek to my grandparents' home. We'd turn silent with carsickness as the journey progressed, stomachs hungry for the roast that we knew was waiting for us on arrival.

We didn't know a huge amount people, nor did my parents. They had some childhood friends, some friends from college and friends made in our local area. That was about it.

Life was spent alongside people at different stages, ages and those with various life experiences. It was clear to see that much of life was a stage, proven by watching those around you move through the challenges of parenting. There was a confidence that you gained from watching others a step or two ahead of you.

You didn't create your own village; your community was the people you saw regularly, and your friends happened to be the ones you chose to spend more time around. You had more people in your life who'd seen you grow from a younger age, seen you develop and known your family over the years.

Extended family were far more likely to be within driving distance. People retired earlier so there may have been more hands to help when needed. People started families younger, so those hands to help were potentially sprightlier. Maternity groups and playgroups weren't a lengthy, varied offering. Nor was it as cheap or as accessible to eat out with children, so more meals were eaten at home and whatever green spaces were nearby were the go-to playgrounds.

Now

I don't know about you, but I know so many people. I know so many people but I don't feel known by many of them. I mean, really known. I could count on one hand the friends I'm still in touch with from childhood and there are contacts in my phone that I'd struggle to tell you how the heck I know them.

We have so many acquaintances, contacts, people we've

collected throughout the various stages and contexts of our lives but how many people really know us? Know how we tick, know our story, know the bumps in the road that have made us *us*. We are having more conversations than ever, in more formats than ever (digital and spoken), yet how much intimacy is there?

Despite the fact that I've never been so connected, at times I've never felt so disconnected and lonely. There is far more sharing than ever, millions of images and words shared every second, but there's less human connection, less intimacy.

> *I used to talk to my friends on the phone loads. But now when I get a phone call, I do anything I can to avoid it. I feel so communicated-out. Even though the hundreds of quick connections I have with people in the day are nowhere near as meaningful as those long chats.*

Anonymous

The increased availability of education and the decrease in job availability means that it is becoming more common for families to become scattered. We take physical steps away from our historic support networks.

At eighteen, I moved to Loughborough, a two-hour motorway trek from my family home. There, I met Tarun, now my husband. After we graduated we moved to London to seek work and further training opportunities. I now live two and a half hours away from my parents. That's a fair drive when you've got a small one or three, who will likely require extra stops, and you can't quite do a daytime round trip, so weekends are ring-fenced instead for our chaos to descend.

We end up trying to cram in memory-making catch-ups and the quality time that would be more scattered throughout days and weeks, if the distance between us wasn't quite so far. I don't doubt that many of you nodding along to this, live further away, maybe even a flight away from family.

These days we are far more likely to have to create our own villages of community. And we are more likely to gravitate to those treading the same paths as us. Most of our friends locally share our life stage. Our kids are similar ages, our challenges are similar, and whilst in many ways it's lovely, we miss out on the rich benefits of our personal communities being multi-generational.

When we don't feel really known, we are less likely to share our internal world. If we are struggling or feeling challenged by something, it can feel overwhelming to provide the relevant back-story to help someone understand where we are coming from. I haven't known many of my local friends for longer than five years.

It's pretty tricky to share a back-story amidst the half-finished sentences of playdates and over the rowdy cacophony of overtired babies and toy-tug-o'-warring toddlers at playgroups. We all relate to the challenges we mutually face: the frustrations that come with relationships stretched by increase in family size and decrease in time to invest in one another, the challenges of family boundaries, bank balances, routines and box ticking.

The worries and challenges that unite us can sometimes feel bigger because we add value and attention to them.

We affirm anxieties in each other, making it feel acceptable to worry about the things that we do. It's great to feel like we aren't alone in this kind of worrying but it shouldn't stop there. Just because it's not uncommon to be anxious as a mum, doesn't mean that we shouldn't be seeking tools, techniques and insights to claim back the headspace taken.

Through being increasingly open about common anxieties, some of the more entrenched, complex challenges get less airtime. This is because many relationships lack the depth, history and opportunities for quality time that enable us to feel safe enough to 'go there'.

Comparison

Then

With far fewer television channels, zero social media and only a shelf of magazines available to buy, the bombardment of shiny portrayals of life wasn't as intense as it is now. Yes, images may have been tweaked, but technology wasn't as advanced.

As a child, finances for my family were challenging to say the least. There were times where money was very tight and many times where we were saved by the selfless generosity of friends and family.

There were times our old car broke down beyond affordable repair and someone would lend us theirs so we could continue the rural school runs. There was the time my sister was in the last stretch of her life and someone booked us a family break that would have otherwise been unaffordable. They gave us the gift of making some final precious memories together.

We had some friends who were financially wealthy. I vividly remember my brother and I being taken to a swimming pool at his health club to give my parents some respite and time to focus on my sister. We entered this gleaming world beyond the local public swimming pool. We were entranced by the polished floors, the bottles of water and fluffy towels there for the taking. It felt luxurious. It cast our lives into fresh perspective and I hungered to return to this different, happier world. I guess, money was the main thing that separated lifestyles.

And I remember having a pretty, petite friend. I went to her house after school one day and we dressed up in her clothes. I threw her top over my head but struggled to get both arms in, as my frame was different. Again, this gave me instant insight of difference and fresh fodder for comparison that the increased exposure to advertising would only work to embed.

In the past, the lives of those around you weren't fed to you in a curated, edited stream; they were real. You saw the rough and the smooth, the highs and the lows. You were less likely to idealise them.

Now

Now? Billion-pound industries thrive from us feeling like we need to be more and to have more. Our economy blooms on us feeling less than others and needing to fill that gap with something ... preferably something we have to pull out the cash for. Can't afford it? No problem, no need to wait. Sign up for a new credit card or open a store card. Happiness is only a signature away.

You don't need something else to be worth something more.

There's an external and internal pressure to have it all and do it all.
Sukriti

We are encouraged to live lives we can't afford, to obtain a happiness that can't be found there. We are bombarded with curated imagery chosen to show life's highlights. We naturally develop a warped sense of what is and should be attainable.

We are more likely to lean into the utter lie that those images are the big and only pictures. No matter how we try to rationalise it, when we're sold a big fib at such consistent volume, it's like trying to plug a leaking dam with scraps of toilet roll.

Social media

Then

Huh? What's that?

Now

Social media arrived on our front door step, banging the hell out of it.

Cherry

Social media is one of the most dominant tools of our generation. It's also undeniably one of the most exciting and innovative advances. It offers communities where there was previously a sense of isolation. But it can also be hugely destructive and addictive. It is a tough one to balance.

There's a whole world of 'more' in the palm of your hand. We scroll, we switch off, but we never stop consuming. Other people's lives, adverts and stories skip past our vision in a constant stream. It's hard to tell what's real and what isn't. We may think it doesn't matter but it does.

We view social media through the filter of our mood. If you are feeling depleted in any way, you're going to be more vulnerable to comparison as it's harder to access your rational brain. You're likely to come away feeling more of what you were already feeling.

I've just done two years of pastoral care in secondary school and the impact of social media and reality TV programmes is undeniable. Even as an adult I forget that 'gram life' isn't always real life.

Anonymous

Standards and expectations are higher when comparing ourselves to what we see of others. We start to shut out our messier bits, both online and offline. We have started to believe that we are only acceptable or loveable in our best state. We're all sharing so much more, but the temptation to share less of our authentic selves perpetuates this cycle.

On occasions, a mindless scroll through social media has left me feeling educated and less alone. But more often, seeing the exciting, fulfilled lives of hundreds of others feels like salt on the wounds of my vulnerability and I leave feeling worse.

When I'm feeling strong and well rested, I am less susceptible to believing that all I see is real, and that not every mum is creating Instagram-worthy crafts or sandwiches shaped like bunnies or has a freezer full of lovingly homemade cubes of weaning delights. Or that every other woman in their mid-thirties seems to iron their clothes, and their kids smile and bake and don't fight over the same sodding toy all the flippin' time (even though you relented and bought them one each).

We're more anxious because we are more aware of all the small seemingly insignificant parts of people's lives. Before we didn't know exactly how tidy someone's utility room was or the details of what our work colleagues had got up to at the weekend. But now we know all these things and we feel the pressure to make our houses the cleanest, our social lives the most exciting, our relationships the most perfect etc. This, on top of all the other pressures we had before, just piles up. It's something I'm trying to be really conscious of.

Leila

With my rational brain weakened by chronic sleep deprivation after having Charlie, I fell prey to the supermum myth. I felt I had to portray life in a way that didn't match the truth of my experience. I had to smile when I felt dark and alone. I had to speak of love for my new baby, when I felt disconnection.

I felt like a failure because what I believed I 'should' be experiencing was far from my own truth. The images bombarding my eyeline only set this belief in concrete and fed my anxiety like petrol thrown onto a fire. Only when I started to shrug off my weakening façade could light start to seep into the dark places.

Comparison stops us enjoying the richness of life that we do have. It tells us that happiness can't truly be found where we are.

Conclusion

Our full, fast lives contribute to the general increase in anxiety of our generation. My hope is that you have a greater insight into why mothering in our generation can feel so pressured and anxiety provoking. We need to go gently on ourselves. There's enough external pressure on us as mums. When we apply it internally too, it's no wonder we sometimes feel we may snap.

I asked my social media followers whether they felt we were a more anxious generation and why? The overwhelming response was that social media and the consistently distorted reality we are fed has a huge impact on our mental health. It makes me want to monitor my social media usage in an attempt to protect myself from this double-edged sword. The world in the palm of our hand never sleeps. Culture will feed anxiety but, with awareness, we can choose how we interact with it.

Top Tip

If you're feeling particularly vulnerable to comparison, consider your social media usage.

JOURNAL POINTS

- Are there any areas of your lifestyle that might be fuelling your anxiety?
- Can you make any tweaks that might address this?
- How much of your life is filtered?
- What is your main concern about being more authentic?

Chapter 5

What makes you feel anxious?

Mantra: *I am worth a life punctuated with
good experiences.*

Can you recall a more carefree time in your life where everything seemed a bit simpler? Perhaps your anxiety just crept up on you alongside the increase of responsibilities and pressures. Or maybe it was triggered by a specific life event. In this chapter, we are going to consider when and why your anxious thoughts became harder to shrug off.

When we begin to identify the things that have instigated or worsened our anxiety, and question what purpose it serves us, we can address it more specifically. You may identify with one or more of the potential causes of your anxiety. I can reassure you that it's normal for there to be a combination of factors present. I'm going to start by talking you through the things that have impacted mine.

When did I start to worry or feel anxious like this?

My journey

I'm not sure when the anxiety crept in for me. Our family dynamics have always edged on the challenging side of things. The biggest life event for me was when my younger sister was diagnosed with a brain tumour at the age of four.

I was suddenly made aware, at the tender age of seven, of the gossamer-thin line we walked upon between life and death. And how life's curveballs could come, seemingly out of nowhere, to whisk you off your carefree perch and leave you feeling like the bottom of the world had fallen out. Life went from feeling safe, to being an uncertain place.

I remember sitting in the waiting room awaiting my sister's prognosis. My parents sat ashen-faced on the tethered plastic waiting-room chairs. I wanted so desperately for life to be OK. I felt like we were teetering on the edge of a precipice. I felt like we were all going to fall over.

Perhaps it was in that moment where I felt a burning desperation, wanting to stop the cruel twist our family life was taking. In my head, on loop, was the music from the album we played at the weekend, when the fire was lit and food was cooking. The music meant comfort. Stability. Mundane, beautiful, boring.

I suddenly yearned for boring more than ever.

Writing is therapeutic. I've written that out, and now I've identified the moment my eyes opened to the fact that, ultimately, I don't have the control I want to have. I know this all sounds foreboding but it's helpful to identify that *this* is what anxiety is. Anxiety is the stark awareness of the fragility of life and lack of control where we really want it.

Anxiety is the stark awareness of the fragility of life and lack of control where we really want it.

Here are some anxious thoughts I've had in the last couple of days:

- *Charlie is going to have an asthma attack and die before I can pick up his new inhaler.*
- *I'm going to crash the car with the kids in it.*
- *My husband is going to get hit by a drunk driver whilst walking back late from the pub with friends.*
- *My parents are coming tonight and they'll die in a car crash.*
- *My headache is cancer, like my sister's. It must run in the family.*
- *I'm too tired to give my husband much attention. Therefore, he'll probably have an affair.*
- *People won't like this book or find it as helpful as I deeply hope they may.*
- *I'm juggling too much, I can't do anything well. I'm a failure.*

All these thoughts touch on a sense of lack of control. All these thoughts sound like statements of truth or they race ahead into a future that hasn't yet happened. And all of these thoughts are possibilities, right? You can't promise me that they won't happen. It's not like I'm considering an alien invasion or monsters under my bed. My mind is throwing me possible outcomes.

Some of those thoughts came to me at 2 a.m. after being awoken by Charlie, who had stirred to discover that his bedroom door was 1.786° more shut than it was when he fell asleep (apparently this is *not* OK). Each of those anxious thoughts could have easily had me spiralling into a whirlwind of anxiety. They certainly used to.

Sleep would be incredibly hard to come by once I'd considered any of these scenarios for more than a fleeting moment. Those whirlwind spirals, like that horrible kind of dream you're always relieved to wake up from, the ones that take your heart time to slow, and you may need to turn on a light to reassure yourself that it wasn't real all along. The thoughts will come, but it's what we do with them that matter.

So those have been some of my triggers for anxiety, now let's explore what some of yours may be.

Looking at your circumstantial triggers

These are the life events that have us feeling out of control and suddenly aware of all the things that can go wrong. They are usually events in which we've felt scared, helpless or devalued. Some examples might be work stress, grief, illness, loss or relationship breakdown. When we go through emotional distress, the emotions we experienced can be triggered by other situations that are in any way similar.

I lost my mum to cancer when I was young. Whenever my dad gets ill, my anxiety goes wild – even if he says it's a cough, I think it's lung cancer. Then I can't stop checking in on him. He finds it a bit annoying. But I am so scared to lose him too.

Petra

I find my own anxiety triggered when one of my children complains of headaches or if they are driven by someone else (not that I rate my driving that highly but I feel more in control when they are within 'are we nearly there yet' earshot). My mind jumps to assumptions that bad things are going to happen. Often cancer and crashes. Both of which I've experienced. You can't quite scrub things like that off your history.

Sometimes the anxiety we feel is displaced. It's like when you're feeling frustrated with a partner. You haven't managed to talk it through. Instead, you take all your frustration out on the pan you've dropped on the floor. It's not really about the pan. The dropped pan is bearing the brunt of your bigger, triggered feelings of frustration.

Is your anxiety acting as a coping mechanism for you?

I'm going to say something that may sound strange. Anxiety sometimes feels like a coping mechanism that can make us feel safe in times of uncertainty. We can believe that our habit of overthinking about all the things that could go wrong helps us prepare ourselves for those worst-case scenarios.

Imagine that my son has a rash. My first thought is 'Oh, there's a small rash. I'd better keep an eye on it.' Then I recall a devastating

Anxiety sometimes feels like a coping mechanism that can make us feel safe in times of uncertainty.

story about a friend's cousin's son having meningitis. The fear of meningitis suddenly becomes a whirlwind in my mind, terrifying me. I consider, in detail, what would happen if it was meningitis. It suddenly feels like a very real threat, so I cancel all playdates so that I can watch him closely.

Thinking everything through makes me feel purposeful, like I'm preparing myself for the worse to happen. I believe I'll be more likely to spot meningitis because I've lived through the whole experience in my own head. Also, if it was meningitis, then I feel I'm more prepared for the onslaught of emotion that would come with it.

I feel silly saying this but worrying kind of makes me feel useful. I feel like at least I'm thinking about the situation a lot so I'm kind of preparing myself in case something happens. It is quite tiring though and it doesn't actually gain anything really, I know that.

Anonymous

It's undeniable that anxiety helps us consider the possibilities. However, the challenge comes when we take it further than a simple consideration and start to imagine and live through the dreadful possibilities in our mind. In doing that, we unnecessarily put ourselves through feelings of fear, grief, loss, helplessness or hopelessness.

I don't doubt that every member of my family played out in their minds the loss of my sister before she died. Imagining the heartache and emptiness. But when it did happen, the fact that we'd lived through some of it in our imaginations did nothing to protect or lessen the reality when it did happen. We had lived it more times than we'd needed to.

The thing is, when our resources are challenged in any way, as they often are in these early months and years of caring for our children, we move from the rational to the irrational much faster. Rationalising requires energy. Unless you're getting a solid night of sleep and aren't depleted in any way, you probably don't possess an overflowing abundance of energy.

Anxiety isn't a suitable coping mechanism for us. It's exhausting in so many ways, emotionally, physically and mentally. If you recognise that it has become a way of coping for you, then you're in the right place amidst the pages of this book.

Were you taught to be anxious?

It may be that through childhood you've learnt that anxious thoughts are a way to process difficult situations. Perhaps someone in your life had a habit of verbalising worst-case scenarios when someone was unwell or when faced with uncertainty or fear.

My mum was definitely a glass-half-empty kind of person. She was always saying the negatives of everything. As soon as I was old enough to drive, she assumed I'd crash and she'd want me to call her to tell her I arrived at my friend's house, even if it was only ten minutes away. I feel like I've got that habit now. Just always thinking of the worst things that might happen. I kind of want to learn to be more positive as I don't want Jack to feel like this.

Jacqui

After living through my sister's brain tumour, I remember my dad studying my pupils when I complained of a headache. I could sense his anxiety spike as he feared that he'd lose another daughter. So now I try to calm my mind and its racing thoughts when my children complain of headaches.

You may have had a parent or carer who fixated on worst-case scenarios or consistently focused on the negatives of life's circumstances. Maybe you were closely exposed to someone who used controlling or obsessive behaviour to deal with difficult emotions in pursuit of a sense of regaining control.

I lived with my aunt. She would check the front door so many times before we left. I do the same now. I can't really help it. I have this thing where I can't believe I've actually locked it and that someone is going to break in.

Anonymous

We had a close family friend who feared crashing the car, so, as a result, she never drove despite having a licence. Whilst this is such a common anxiety, perhaps it fuelled my own driving anxiety later on in life. She modelled that if you were really scared of something, the best thing to do was to avoid it.

In an ideal world, parents and authority figures would teach us how to deal with stress in a constructive way. Instead we may be taught to live fearfully or defensively, causing a higher level of stress and that heightened on-edge feeling we are familiar with.

Don't despair, though. As we become aware of these traits, things can start to change. When a behaviour is learned, with work, time and the right support, it can be unlearned. Obviously, it takes a while for our new way of coping to become our default, so it's important to be patient with yourself. It's not a quick fix, but I promise you it's worth the investment of your time and energy.

Considering physical triggers of your anxiety

Have you had a health check recently? I bet your baby has had a fair few. As mothers, our attention is so focused on our children's wellbeing that it's easy to neglect our own. It's amazing how much more likely we are to be proactive when it's someone we love. I'd like you to extend some of that attentiveness to yourself.

Don't forget that you've undergone some mountainous hormonal shifts that take a while to settle into a rhythm. Therefore, if physical symptoms of anxiety are bothering you it can be helpful to rule out underlying causes.

Honestly, now I've had a baby, I notice my hormones so much more. I don't know if it's because I'm tired but my anxiety gets so much worse before I get my period. Now I've worked out that it happens, I can put it down to hormones, which helps. I never noticed it before.

Sabine

A doctor can also consider any medications that could be exacerbating or mimicking any physical feelings of anxiety. Chronic illness or changes in medication can also make someone feel anxious. It's beneficial to get a check-up should you have any concerns in case something needs to be addressed.

There are other external things that can spark physical feelings that mimic anxiety. The spikes that caffeine and sugar can give us are a good example. That heightened, buzzing feeling, for some, can be very reminiscent of anxiety.

I've had many clients in the past who came to me complaining of feeling on edge. After a bit of exploration, we discovered that the numerous teas and coffees containing heaped spoons of sugar were the likely cause. When we physically feel anxious, it can trigger anxious thoughts and vice versa. For some, the physical effects of exercise can also trigger anxiety, as the increased heart rate and any resulting light-headedness can blur the line between what is anxiety and what is a common physical response to exertion.

Pay attention to the things that put your body under stress.

I've had clients say that they can't exercise because it makes them anxious but once we've identified this, they are more able to make the distinction. Feelings of anxiety, regardless of how they are triggered, can quickly spiral without the correct tools and insight, because the feelings themselves can trigger further anxiety.

Pay attention to the things that put your body under stress, such as exhaustion, sleep deprivation, dehydration and hunger. These are all too common states we find ourselves in as mothers of a new baby.

We are far less likely to meet and be attentive to our own physical needs, putting the body under stress and increasing cortisol levels (the stress hormone). Only yesterday, after spending an entire day on the go, did I have a wave of feeling stressed, irritable and spaced-out. It suddenly occurred to me that I had eaten only a hastily shoved-down banana, chased by two cups of tepid coffee ... it was now 3 p.m. I refuelled and glugged a pint of water and things shifted physically and mentally.

What happens when your anxiety is fuelled by trauma?

Trauma is a negative event (but can also be a series of events over time) that for whatever reason causes an intense feeling of fear and lack of safety. Due to the intensity of fear experienced at the time, the event isn't correctly processed and stored by the brain.

It's like dropping your sunglasses. You pick them up to find them cracked and scratched, right down the middle of the lenses. You put them back on, but now, instead of seeing things as they are, scratches distort your vision as you try to peer through.

I went through birth trauma and felt a bit neglected. So for a few months, whenever I was feeling emotional it really panicked me out when I was on my own. I would call my husband and want him to come home which wasn't possible. I'm not sure what I was scared about. I got some therapy and it's really helped. Being alone took me back to the delivery room and how I felt then.

Alysia

It might be that you've experienced physical or emotional abuse, grief or bullying, or perhaps you've had a traumatic incident such as a physical or emotional breakdown, a difficult birth, a car crash or dangerous experience in the past. Past trauma can rear its head when our usual defences and coping mechanisms are challenged by the life shift, tiredness and hormonal fluctuations that come with the postpartum period.

If you've undergone trauma or sustained stress of any kind, it may trigger or intensify anxious feelings and thoughts. When I talk about trauma, I don't only mean moments in which you've feared for your life, I mean any experience you've experienced as traumatic. I say 'you' because we all experience things differently due to our own unique histories, personalities, ways of processing overwhelming emotions and the coping mechanisms we employ afterwards.

Not everyone who experiences what may be perceived as a traumatic event will become psychologically traumatised.

An example of trauma

One of my clients came to me to discuss her experience of giving birth. She'd had what would be considered a text-book labour with no emergency intervention. Her labour wasn't too long and she had been administered the pain relief she'd requested. Her baby had been born healthy and she was discharged the next day.

However, my client had found the birth terrifying. She'd felt out of control of her own body and was experiencing flashbacks of the pushing stage and having regular night-mares. She'd been pep-talking herself into believing that because her birth was straightforward, it wasn't justified that she should feel this way.

My client had devalued her feelings because she didn't feel 'should' feel traumatised. She told me that some of her friends had far more medically challenging births and yet seemed OK. On exploring this further, we discovered that her grandmother had died during childbirth, and whilst at the time she hadn't made this link, she felt out of control and vulnerable, fearing her own death. With this insight, we could then begin to help her process the feelings and fears in a way that would slowly lessen the symptoms of trauma.

It's important that you don't diminish any experience of trauma by comparing it to other people's experiences. Your experience isn't comparable, no matter how similar it may seem. And when we diminish it, we're more likely to avoid seeking the support we need and deserve.

My experiences of trauma

After my traumatic postpartum experience with Charlie's undiagnosed silent reflux, a rough night with Florence had me panicking that it was happening again. There were mornings I'd be in an almost inconsolable state of fear.

Tiredness impacted my ability to easily access my rational brain and reassure myself. Despite Florence not showing signs of reflux, any obvious discomfort would trigger my fear response.

There were times, when considering having a third child, my decision was influenced by fear of a repeat of what was the hardest year of my life. The traumatised part of me wanted to protect myself from experiencing that again. It told me that perhaps we should stop at two children.

I experienced a wave of fear whenever I saw someone with a crying baby and a wave of jealousy when I saw someone with a content one. I had to process some of the trauma and put in place a strategy that would help me cope should we go through something similar again. On doing this, I felt able (albeit nervous), to consider trying for a third child. I'm glad the trauma didn't win. It would have robbed me of experiencing the joy of my little girl.

I didn't drive for a decade due to being impacted by the trauma of being in a car crash at eighteen years old. I bumbled along for years using buses, walking miles and being driven by my husband. However, I remember the day I found myself pushing a hefty, shopping-laden buggy up a steep hill, in pouring rain, on a three-mile round trip to a friend's house. My car at home, gathering dust. I realised how much my fear was impacting my day-to-day life. I finally addressed it and now it feels like my world has opened up.

Addressing my fear meant I could invest in certain friendships and take the kids on days out. Yes, I still get waves of anxiety as I overtake lorries on the motorway or drive down country lanes reminiscent of the one I crashed on but I have faithful techniques to help me ride those waves. Most importantly, I am no longer a prisoner of fear, held within a walkable radius. It was tough to address, it took energy and tentative steps outside my comfort zone. But it was worth it.

If you've experienced trauma, there is hope

Your trauma doesn't have to impact your life in this way forever. I will share techniques to help you regain a sense of safety. However, regardless of how much your trauma impacts your daily life, therapy has the aim of helping your mind process what you've been through. When we have unprocessed trauma, it's like we are still living it a bit in our day-to-day life. It can easily impact the decisions we make and our ability to enjoy things.

Trauma fuels anxious and intrusive thoughts.

There are many symptoms of trauma, so please consult your doctor or therapist in order to gain specific clarification. Processing trauma allows it to slowly slot back into our past in less of a spiky, painful way. If you're looking for a therapist, search for someone specialising in trauma, using techniques such as The Rewind Technique or EMDR (eye movement desensitisation and reprocessing).

Unprocessed trauma fuels anxiety because it's a constant reminder that bad things can happen. Because you've experienced the psychological repercussions, you know how painful those feelings can be, so you are likely to go to further lengths to avoid them.

You are worth finding the resources and space to process your trauma. Trauma is worth addressing because often, in trying to protect and defend ourselves from the possibility of pain, we can also end up protecting ourselves from good experiences too. You are worth a life punctuated with good experiences and memories.

Getting to the bottom of it

I hope this chapter has helped you identify some of the causes of your anxiety. Understanding where it may have originated can enable you to seek more specific support and tools, and hopefully cultivate more kindness towards yourself. If you didn't relate to any of the possible causes I mention here, that's OK. It might just take a bit more exploration through therapy.

Top Tip

Address your caffeine, alcohol and sugar intake if you feel it might be exacerbating your anxiety.

JOURNAL POINTS

- Can you think back to when you first recognised your anxiety. What was happening in your life?
- What do you feel has triggered or is triggering your anxiety?

▶

- Is there anything that exacerbates your anxiety in your lifestyle or puts your body under stress?
- What steps might you take to help take some pressure off yourself?
- Do you believe you are worth good experiences and feelings?
- Would you benefit from trauma therapy? If so, explore what the options may be for you.

Chapter 6

How do you cope with your anxiety?

Mantra: *Addressing my anxiety and worry allows my world to grow.*

Now we have explored the foundations of anxiety, we are going to look at the different ways you may have dealt with anxious feelings and thoughts. We implement mechanisms as a way of trying to cope with or control anxiety. It's completely natural to want to lessen the impact that it has on your mind and life. However, often these coping mechanisms don't actually lessen the anxiety, they simply hide it for a while. They are like the fancy bottle of wine that tastes glorious from the glass but takes 'headache revenge' in the morning.

In this chapter, we are going to explore lots of common coping mechanisms. Identifying them gives you the opportunity to address them and then implement some new mechanisms that will help support your mental health in a really positive way, rather than hinder you.

Avoiding the issue

On a recent trip to the coast, full of hormones and with eye bags telling of a week of broken sleep, I kept having intrusive thoughts of tossing Florence into the sea. It sounds horrifying, and whilst I knew I wouldn't throw my scrumptious lady into the ocean, the thoughts came and went like the tide.

What I could have (and previously would have) done, to avoid these thoughts, would have been to either take another route or walked on the other side of the road from the beautiful coastal path. I'd have listened to those thoughts, pondered on them, felt that fear rise and made sure I did whatever I could to avoid the trigger for those intrusive thoughts, which was in this case – the coastal path.

> *I felt so anxious about Jenson choking when we began weaning, that he ate smooth purée until he was one. If he ever gagged, I panicked, so I avoided all lumps.*
>
> Jenny

There are so many ways we can avoid our triggers. I didn't drive for a full ten years due to the intrusive thoughts about crashing and dying that skipped into my mind as I, white-knuckled, gripped the wheel. When I did finally start driving again out of necessity, I would feel a panic attack rising on the motorway and would pull off at the first opportunity to swap seats with my husband. Being behind the wheel was a trigger, getting away from it allowed the angry, swelling wave of anxiety to return to a still sea.

How avoidance doesn't serve you

Avoidance is a natural, inbuilt mechanism to avoid things that make us feel fearful, uncomfortable or in pain. However, this mechanism goes into overdrive when we perceive something as a far larger threat than it is.

If I'd listened to those anxious thoughts on that coastal path, I wouldn't have been able to breathe in that fresh salty air. I wouldn't have witnessed the boys' delight at the boats or their small pointing fingers as they named the colours of the bobbing buoys. Sweet memories I wouldn't have made.

If I'd avoided driving forever, I would feel marooned on our development. I would have had to negotiate three kids on the bus that rarely runs. We would have missed out on playdates, trips and doctor's appointments. When we avoid our triggers, we limit our experience of life. Whilst it sure feels safer, it makes our worlds smaller.

Every time we avoid our trigger, we give it authority. Imagine if I avoided every tantrum my three-year-old threw by giving him whatever the hell he wanted. The issue would be bigger in the long term. He'd feel pretty authoritative if every time he threatened a tantrum I gave him chocolate or bought him one of those expensive magazines covered in plastic tat.

The more I continued to walk along the coastal path without throwing my daughter in, and the more I drove without being in a fatal accident, the less control those thoughts had. When we avoid our trigger, we miss out on the chance to chip away at the authority it holds. But when we approach the things that trigger us with some good techniques that allow us to ride the wave of anxiety, we grow in confidence.

Imagine anxiety as a wave or a labour surge. It peaks and then falls again. It doesn't continue rising forever. It simply can't. Sometimes those waves of anxiety come as I overtake lorries on the motorway. I use my favourite breathing and grounding techniques to calm my nervous system and I continue. The wave abates and I'm still on the road. An anxious thought might tell me that every drive would end in a fatal crash. By approaching each drive with sturdy tools, I'm able to rationalise that the anxious thought is categorically incorrect.

A health visitor taught me the difference between gagging and choking. I went on a first aid course so I'd know what to do. I had to talk myself through it when I started giving him proper food but now I'm much more comfortable and he really likes all the different stuff he eats. He's also putting on weight.

Jessica

Isolating ourselves

The next coping mechanism we are going to identify is that of isolation. I remember a few weeks after Florence was born, I was in that flurry of 'How do I do this?' I had invited a good friend to come over and meet our new addition. I woke feeling floored and tearful. I texted her an hour before and told her not to come over because I was a mess. My text message literally read something like, 'Hey Barbara. Don't come over, I'm a mess.' I felt low, so my coping mechanism was to retreat.

I've got a few friends who go quiet when they are struggling. Messages go unanswered, opportunities to meet up go excused. Some of us shut down and lock up when we feel low, when the opposite would be most helpful.

> *When I get overly worried or anxious, I shut down. I keep my thoughts private as I worry people will think I'm mad. What can they do to help anyway? It's lonely, actually.*
>
> Anonymous

I'm not talking about those times you need a bit of downtime to regroup. Those can be so helpful. My antenatal friends and I would call them 'lockdown days'. They were an opportunity to take things slower, chuck on a hoodie and hunker down with a movie and snacks. They might have come during a baby's growth spurt, teething days or following a run of rough nights. These days aren't born out of a desire to shut off and protect yourself from the world. They are a recognition of a need to refuel so that you can go back out into it.

Isolation is that hedgehog reaction. You may use it when the going gets tough and you fancy curling up like a hedgehog into a small, spiky ball. The aim is to protect yourself from engaging with the world around you and the emotions inside you.

How isolation doesn't serve you

I don't know about you, but when I isolate myself, my thoughts get bigger and louder. When we shut off from others physically, there are fewer reassuring voices and familiar faces to ground us. We need other people to balance us sometimes, to offer different insights, energy, moods, words and acts of support.

One of the best things I did during the early days of motherhood was to ensure I connected with at least one other adult each day, and left the house once per day. Whether I picked up the phone, met someone for coffee or went to a baby sensory class. Sometimes I had to push myself, especially when feeling flat and shattered. But whether it was a phone call or a brisk walk, I always felt perked up by the fresh air and the company.

My whirlwinds of thought can get darker in the night when everything is quiet. Do you ever have a bad dream and turn the light on to help you shake off the feelings? Seeking the right company and social interaction when the temptation is to hedgehog can feel like switching on a light after being stirred by a bad dream.

We isolate ourselves out of the desire to keep our world smaller and to feel safer. If we do less and encounter less, we risk less. However, we also end up missing out on life and positive social experiences. If you find yourself wanting to isolate, consider what you might be trying to protect yourself from. Is there a friend or family member you can text or call who has been historically supportive?

I'd find myself cancelling playdates and stuff last minute. Especially if there were going to be people I didn't know. It kind of made my social anxiety worse because I started going less and I started to feel really lonely. I realised I needed to break the barrier, so I would ask a friend to meet me before, kind of like a comfort blanket. I built my confidence back up after that and now I only get butterflies before I arrive.

Kira

Putting on a mask

This is one of my go-to coping mechanisms. During the depths of my postnatal anxiety, I remember walking into town. I was pushing the double buggy in the sunshine, wearing shorts and oversized sunglasses. Anyone passing by would have seen a mum striding purposefully with her two under two. It would have been understandable for onlookers to assume I was thriving in my new role.

It was a mask. Only fifteen minutes before, I had cried desperately on the phone to my husband saying, 'I can't do this.' Mascara streamed down my face as I took sharp gulps of air. I felt like a guilty, undeserving failure of a mother. Then I dried my eyes and put on a (rather high pitched) happy voice for the kids. On went another layer of water-proof mascara, some huge sunglasses to hide the hive-like blotches. I headed out into the sunshine to a playgroup.

For me, putting on the mask of having it all together, was a defence against falling apart. Don't we all do this sometimes? When we utter 'I'm fine', during the times we're actually not hugely OK. Maybe we want to avoid judgement or we don't wish to talk or think about how we really feel. Being vulnerable is an admission that we need the support, comfort, guidance or empathy of others, and sometimes that feels like a big step to take.

> *When I'm having a tough day, I actually think I smile more. It's not because I'm actually happy, it's because I really don't want to talk about it and if people see someone looking happy, they don't bother asking questions.*
>
> Leah

How putting on a mask doesn't serve you

Putting on a mask is a protective mechanism, like raising a shield in a battle. It can serve a purpose at times, protecting us and enabling us to find strength in challenging circumstances. A shield is valuable in battle. But if the soldier continued holding his raised shield after the attacking swords had been thrown down, he'd be defending himself unnecessarily.

Wearing your mask when you don't need to is a form of emotional isolation. It keeps people out, and keeps your feelings unspoken and unvalued. It's OK not to tell everyone everything. It's a privilege and an honour for those you choose to lower your shield for. Not everyone wins the right to see into your inner life but it's so important for your mental health that you let some see beyond the mask.

On Oscar's first day at school, I found the school and nursery run with three so stressful. In fact, I don't think I actually breathed for an hour. I was invited for coffee with about fifteen mums who didn't really know one another. I arrived, sat down and told the mums at my table that I had raging hormones and found my first school run experience so stressful. Old me would have been mortified to share such honest insight with strangers but it immediately gave the others licence to be honest about their experiences too. It cut through the small talk, and I felt I could be myself. It can become quite liberating.

Wearing your mask when you don't need to is a form of emotional isolation.

Often the more complex my feelings are, the more tempting it is to shove on the mask and be done with it. I'm happier talking about stress, social anxiety and hormones than I am my feelings of inadequacy that stem from childhood. Not everyone needs to know everything.

When we do take our masks down for a select few, it can strengthen those relationships and make us feel heard. It can also help us untangle them, introducing valuable perspective. For those select few, it's an honour to be let in. Not everyone deserves the insight into your inner life, especially if they have previously taken advantage of your vulnerability. Being let close to the parts that you find hard to reveal is a privilege.

Dropping our mask is about taking small steps and risks with authenticity and vulnerability. It's important that we feel safe and heard even if that person doesn't fully understand what we're experiencing. Drop that mask a few inches each time until you feel safe to reveal more.

Pretending I was OK the whole time actually made me so tired. I first opened up to another mum friend, totally on impulse. She was so lovely. Then I told my husband that I was struggling with anxiety. I used to think, 'What can anyone else do to actually help me?' But speaking about it took it out of my head and made it feel less heavy. I knew that even if I faked it around other friends, I could be honest with those two.

Leona

Comparing ourselves

We often compare our circumstances with those of others, whether work life or personal life. We do this for numerous reasons. It might calm us or it might make things worse. If Florence has a high temperature, to calm myself, I might recall a friend's child who had a fever with her cold. But I could also recall a situation in which a fever had been a symptom of a rare and fatal illness. Instead of treating Florence's temperature as something I need to address, I'm using other people's circumstances as a guide for how I should feel and react to mine.

I would watch other mums in the street. Everyone looked like they were happy and coping. I felt like the only one who was struggling, it made me feel so ashamed.

Anonymous

We may use comparison to validate and/or shut down our feelings. We can berate ourselves because we are finding things more challenging than someone else. Would you say to the trainee doctor, yawning with their tired, red-rimmed eyes midway through a nightshift, 'What are you complaining about? You're not exactly a heart surgeon. Now, *they* deserve to be tired.'

We may use comparison to validate and/or shut down our feelings.

We acknowledge that with each exam studied for, each life saved, each death processed comes an uncomfortable stretching of capacity. An increasing ability to cope with shifts, traumas, medical mysteries. Only through experience does thinking become quicker, drug calculations become more fluid and reactions become more instinctive.

We value the doctor at every step of training, because they are useful. So why shouldn't we also value ourselves? We are growing as we go, stretching beyond our previous capacities, constantly learning. Growth is life-changing and uncomfortable. Sometimes I feel like I experience a growth spurt as I've pushed through one of those days where I thought I couldn't. Sometimes growth is slow but steady.

It's unfair of me to compare myself, as a mum of three, to my younger self as a mum of one and say, 'I don't know what I was complaining about back then.' We grow as we go. We come with unique histories that dictate we will all experience everything differently. There will always be someone who has it harder or sadder than you, easier and breezier than you.

How comparison doesn't serve you

Comparison is ultimately a desire to validate our feelings, actions or emotions so that they feel justified. The issue is that, as a result, we come off better than someone else, or worse. We give comparison a lot of clout when we use it to tell us whether we're doing a good job or not, or whether our feelings are valid or not.

> *I had a miscarriage with my first baby at six weeks. I was absolutely broken but then a friend told me she'd lost hers at fourteen weeks. I felt like I shouldn't be sad because her situation was much harder. I kind of swallowed down my sadness for ages. Now I realise that we all have a right to feel sad at any pregnancy loss. It's always loss of a dream and a hope in your head. It's the community online that has helped me realise that.*
>
> Anonymous

Next time you find yourself comparing your experience, feelings or acts with someone else's, it's good to think about what you are hoping to have affirmed. It's likely that you believe something about yourself and are looking for external confirmation. We will always find what we're looking for if we look for it long enough.

I believe a lot of what I think. I don't love to think that I might be wrong about myself. If I feel like I'm failing, I'm far more likely to fixate on those who seem like they are thriving as mums, in order to confirm my sense of failure. But still, it doesn't mean that our beliefs about ourselves are true. That's why it's so important to cultivate and invest in our sense of self-worth and inner dialogue.

Comparison only makes us feel better and validated superficially. It's a bit like a drug, we seek another fix when we look at external things to tell us whether we're OK or not. We end up on a rollercoaster of emotion dependent on what we conclude. By comparing our emotional responses and circumstances, we are less likely to process them constructively. We are less likely to give ourselves permission to feel very valid feelings such as frustration, hurt, grief, pride or happiness.

Reliance on substances

When I downloaded Instagram in 2014 I loved the escapism it offered during night feeds. I delighted at the voyeuristic glimpse into the lives of others. The shiny filtered images sat beside honest and raw captured moments. Communities sat in my hands, meeting every single interest no matter how obscure. I found wisdom, humour and comfort.

I also found bountiful 'send coffee' posts. There were dinnertime gin admissions, tales of chocolate bars inhaled behind cupboard doors and prosecco-fuelled playdates. It quickly normalised the desire for sugar highs and rewards sipped from glasses. When it seems that everyone is doing the same thing, we are less likely to reflect on whether it's right for us too.

When I got together with my antenatal friends, everyone would be talking about having a drink over bath time. The stressful part of the day where everyone is overtired. It felt like everyone was doing it. It was like a ritual.

Bea

I know the feeling. Kids down, floor half-heartedly cleared of its assault-course debris, legs tired and shoulders tense. I don't have time to wind down. I have ninety minutes to tidy, answer emails, make dinner and prepare the next day's packed lunches.

I manage to eat the majority of a family-size bag of crisps without noticing and sip a glass of wine each time I bypass the kitchen. The wine is a hug, from the inside out, promising swift anaesthetic to the stress. I mean, it's still there but it's further away, like an echo.

There are many supposedly quick fixes available to us, whispering that they will take the edge off stress or that exhausting, heightened buzz of anxiety – drugs, prescription medication or a cheeky cigarette that transports you to a more carefree decade. And there are many communities that will normalise it for you.

How reliance on substances isn't serving you

It's common to turn to substances of some sort when we want to change feelings. We might desire calm, energy, escapism or sleep instead of anxiety, stress, loneliness, frustration or grief. However, not only are these substances addictive, whilst they might *feel* like they're helping, they are often making it worse. Let's look at our culture's most common and socially acceptable substances: alcohol, sugar and caffeine.

Whilst alcohol feels like a relaxant, regular use adjusts our brain chemistry, decreasing levels of mood-regulating serotonin. It compromises our immune system, slows our brain response and inhibits our judgement and reasoning abilities. Plus, sugar and caffeine, along with many illegal drugs, mimic some of the physical and psychological feelings of anxiety.

Whilst the things we may turn to feel like they fulfil a need for a short while, there's some kind of hangover, whether you are conscious of it or not. A brain chemistry kick-back. A sugar low, a stab of guilt, a caffeine crash, an anxiety spike. And that adds to the pile of things we anaesthetise the next time.

All day, I'd chase a coffee with another coffee because I was so tired. It made my heart go crazy and I'd be really jittery. Looking back, it definitely made my anxiety worse as my body felt so on-edge, and then my head would think so fast too.

Lola

It's healthy and helpful to consider how the things you reach for interact with your mental health. When we're informed, we can make informed decisions that can positively impact the way we feel.

Opting to switch the quick fix for something more beneficial requires conscious effort. This is because the reward comes quickly when we eat or drink something in response to our emotions. We need to be intentional in replacing it with something more beneficial, such as meditation, talking to a friend, having a bath or doing some exercise.

Initially it can be challenging to feel the feelings we'd usually anaesthetise. We feel the stress, the regret, the frustration, the resentment or the anxiety. When we allow ourselves to experience these feelings, we are addressing them rather than suppressing them. We see them for what they are. They are feelings that move and swell like the tide, rather than something that needs to be kept in a dark corner forever. Whilst ten minutes practising mindfulness in place of a stress-fuelled sugar high may take more effort, it doesn't have the same emotional or physical hangover. In fact it makes positive changes to your brain chemistry.

When we allow ourselves to experience these feelings, we are addressing them rather than suppressing them.

I am very partial to using a glass of wine to relax and this is something I've been giving more thought to recently, opting to increase my alcohol-free days. I've been switching my wind-down beverage with a ten-minute stretching or yoga video. I swap out the crisps for herbal tea and a handful of nuts. It doesn't hit the same spot in that very moment but I feel much better for it in the end.

Get to know your body and your mind. Note down what circumstances and emotions leave you reaching for your favourite anaesthetic. Perhaps it's tantrums, traffic, teething or arguments with a partner? Note how long these feelings last before they abate. I know that my hour of need is

7.30–8.30 p.m. If I can ride that out, then the feelings abate and I'm more relaxed.

Challenge yourself to choose something that lowers your heart rate and blood pressure rather than raises them. Seek a replacement that increases your happy hormones rather than inhibits them. It can be helpful to take note of what needs you are trying to meet and what feelings you want to numb through the behaviour and find a more loving way to meet them. Hopefully, as you experience the benefits, you'll feel motivated to make further swaps.

If you want to make changes but are struggling to do so, or they feel addictive, it's worth speaking with a therapist or counsellor. It may be that the feelings you are trying not to feel are complex or historical and would benefit from further insight.

Keeping busy

To deal with anxiety, some of us like to drown it out by keeping busy. Busyness is another way of keeping our minds occupied to distract ourselves from how we really feel. Motherhood is conducive to this in many ways and it's very easy to hop quickly from one appointment to a playdate, to a house chore, to a feed, barely pausing for breath.

Sometimes we fear that if we slow down, the feelings will overwhelm us and we won't be able to gather ourselves again. It is encouraging to remember that feelings can't keep their intensity for long once we start to acknowledge them or process them with the right people.

Finally, perhaps you get a sense of validation through being busy and feeling purposeful. If so, it is common to feel like your sense of worth is being challenged when you slow down.

> *I definitely keep busy on purpose. I know when I must be feeling sad or anxious because I end up doing more stuff to fill up the time. My feelings all come out at night when there's nothing to do or focus on.*
>
> Liz

How keeping busy isn't serving you

As mums, sometimes we're plain busy and it's as simple as that. Life is a juggle and much of the juggle is entirely necessary. Often the best teller of whether you're busy as a form of emotional escape, or just plain busy, is to stop and see what happens. What do you feel?

When you take a break, do you feel anxiety about all the things you need to do? Maybe you feel shattered yet delighted at a chance to stop and refuel. Some of us find that stopping causes us to feel useless, inefficient, scared, lonely or sad.

If I'm totally honest, I get a kick out of being a bit stressed. When I'm juggling lots of balls, I have a spark of adrenaline running through my veins. It makes me feel productive, useful, excited. But it also means I begin to lose sight of how I'm feeling. It means that my internal voice goes less checked and I'm at risk of burnout. I am not a machine. All machines need a break, a service and a refuel to allow them to work safely and efficiently. If not, things begin to fall off, thick metal starts to splinter, they will break. We are no different.

Busyness doesn't touch the underlying issues of anxiety or low sense of worth. It merely covers them up. Because what goes ignored goes unprocessed. When the world becomes merely a blur as we whizz by, we can miss the joy in the small things. I'm reminded of this when I head outside with the kids. They love to plod and don't feel the pull to rush. They are so often distracted by the small things, the bugs, the flowers (and the cigarette butts).

> *I got the flu a couple of years ago. I had such a high temperature and body aches that my mum had to come and look after Danny for me. I didn't do anything for a whole week. I'm such a busy person. I was surprised by how guilty I felt. I couldn't bear feeling so useless.*
>
> Anonymous

Living in this way means our nervous system is more likely to be under stress in the fight or flight state. We are not created to be fully switched on and revved up for a sustained time. It is a protective mechanism but it is not a lifestyle. Stress and anxiety can so easily go hand in hand because, if we don't take time to refuel and realign, we have less energy to rationalise anxious thoughts.

Your value is not the sum of what you do. Your worth isn't based on how efficient you are. Rest isn't uselessness, it's a basic human requirement.

There's more for you

There are so many more coping mechanisms that we could cover here and you may have some more to add. They are simply the things we turn to in order to cope. They often leave a sense of disappointment because they don't fill the gap like we hoped they might. It's like when my three-year-old tries to place a jigsaw piece in the wrong place. It looks right, the image even slightly lines up, but it feels wonky and pushes the other pieces out of alignment.

What started out as a way of helping you feel in control has likely ended up with you feeling controlled. It doesn't have to be this way. When you're aware of how you deal with your anxiety and difficult emotions, you discover that you can choose kinder and more constructive ways to process those feelings.

Top Tip

Imagine anxiety as a wave or a labour surge. It peaks and then falls again.

JOURNAL POINTS

- Which coping mechanisms for your anxiety do you tend to use?
- What feelings do you attempt to meet through using these mechanisms?

▶

- How have these mechanisms served you in the past?
- How have they not served you?
- Which coping mechanism would you most like to address?
- What small step might you take this week in addressing it?

Chapter 7

Looking at personality traits

Mantra: *You are worthy of the compassion you offer to others.*

There's so much to be gained from light-bulb moments in which we make a link between our personality and our behaviour. It provides us with the opportunity to make a tweak that could positively impact our wellbeing, the way we think or the way we experience life.

I'm going to describe some of these different personality traits. These traits are ones I commonly identify in my clients and the mums I speak with.

There's much to be gained from the light-bulb moments in which we make a link between personality and behaviour.

We'll start with the wonderful positives and benefits of those traits and then we'll focus on the challenges they may bring.

You are driven

Let's look at how being a driven person might feed anxiety. I'm quite a driven person. I've done well with work and studies as I tend to be focused and determined. I form habits very quickly and stick to things stubbornly. I learn fast, move fast, juggle many a ball and get lots done. I set an alarm before the kids wake up. Once it resounds, I roll out of bed and into my workout leggings. My husband, however, would be more likely to hit the snooze button.

I'd always be the one asked to do certain tasks because I did them well. I worked in advertising for a few years, helping to manage client accounts. I didn't love the job, but I was thorough and my standards were sky high. Despite disliking it, I was good at it.

Sounds pretty good right? Being driven and motivated can be helpful, until it slips into perfectionism. Perfectionism is exhausting. It's a desire to strive for unattainable standards with ever moving goalposts. After the initial buzz of energy abates, I feel like a plodding donkey with a carrot of perfectionism dangling in front of its head. The prize is tantalisingly close, yet never within reach.

I feel so much pressure to do everything right. But I can't. And then I feel like I've failed at everything when really, I haven't.

Harry

Just because you can do many things, you don't need to do everything. If you've been praised for your efficiency and standards, then perhaps some of your sense of worth is rooted in what you're able to do. If for any reason you can't reach the standard you dream of, you're likely to feel like a failure. Drive coupled with perfectionism is a perfect recipe for overwhelm and burnout.

Just because you can do many things, you don't need to do everything.

I juggle a lot of roles in my life and am sometimes praised for being a supermum. I'm not keen on that phrase. It's an unattainable ideal sold to us by the media, telling us that we can do it all. Yes, I can juggle balls but it comes with a cost. I get tired, irritable and resentful. My husband will confirm, it's not pretty.

New hobbies fall by the wayside if I can't perform to the standard I hope to, at the speed I want to. I have a cupboard full of the ghosts of fleeting hobbies: crochet hooks, Pilates bibles, calligraphy pens. I'd simply rather not do it, than feel like a failure. Procrastination can be something that we perfectionists struggle with because the fear of failure can mean we feel too anxious to even begin something.

Anxiety thrives in places of pressure.

If we apply our drive and perfectionism to motherhood, it's going to provoke anxiety. Our attention is always required in so many different directions. We rarely finish an entire job before being interrupted by a need coming to us from somewhere else: the beep of a washing machine, the ring of a doorbell, the call of the shower, the cry of a hungry baby.

Anxiety thrives in places of pressure. That gap that lies between what we feel we should be doing, achieving and attaining, and what we are *actually* achieving and attaining.

Your value isn't related to how well you do things.

If I get to 7.30 p.m. and I look around to see piles of washing and the kitchen in a state, I feel rubbish. I think, 'What have I done today?' I feel embarrassed when my husband comes home and I haven't brushed my hair. I'm usually so 'together'. He doesn't care though. He sees how full-on things are with a baby, it's just me. I get cross with myself.

Sarah

Bringing balance into being driven

We all struggle, we are all imperfect. That is what makes us human. Notice when you feel that sense of failure creep in. Perhaps you arrived late for something or forgot someone's birthday. Consider the bigger picture, the number of things that your busy, tired mind is trying to juggle.

How would you react to a friend who forgot your birthday amidst the buzz of navigating life with a new baby? Would you want to reassure a friend who felt terrible for turning up late to your house due to an unexpected nappy change? It's easier to find understanding, kindness and forgiveness for others because we often place more value on them than we do on ourselves. You are worthy of the compassion you offer to others.

You like order

It was easy enough to organise and order my life when I was all I had to worry about. Yes, there would be the odd late train or bout of illness that disrupted the rhythm of my days, but, ultimately, I could deal with rare curveballs. Routine and order make me feel safe.

Then I had a baby. And, well, babies don't read the books and get the memos. I hungered for the safe predictability of order in those early weeks and months. My bedside table was piled with books on establishing routines that calmed me and told me that order could be found. I'd plan coffee dates, appointments and journeys down to the minute, to accommodate scheduled nap and wake times.

Sometimes, the sweet spot of order could be found very temporarily. And then along would come growth spurts, teething, weaning, fevers, clock changes, developmental leaps and heatwaves. And as dramatic as it sounds, I felt like the foundations of my sanity had been shaken by a baby group cancellation or an unexpected visitor. My life felt unknown and new, and I needed order to make me feel safe yet it didn't seem to be attainable. Routine was the lifeboat I clung to. But it had a puncture. The more I rely on routine and order to keep me calm, the more likely life's curveballs will trigger anxiety.

I feel myself panicking when I'm at a friend's house and it's near Zed's naptime. It really stresses me out if we're not home in time for him to go down. I don't even know why. Some people seem so chilled about naps and timings.

Zena

Fast-forward a few years and a couple more babies, and I've slowly loosened my grip on my need for strict routine in order to feel grounded. I've had to. Maintaining a sturdy routine for baby Florence has been practically impossible amidst drop-offs, playdates and the constant errands required to run a household. However, I have found it so liberating not to feel anxious if she wakes earlier or sleeps longer than expected. I've had to find other, more consistent and trustworthy ways to feel grounded, such as breathing techniques and small elements of my own routine that I can have more control over. For me this might be ten minutes of daily stretching or my pre-bed routine. It's possible.

Bringing balance into a need for order

Consider what routine means for you. How do you navigate your desire for routine, and the anxiety it provokes when you can't have it? For me, I've found it helpful to recognise when my anxiety was being triggered. For example, I remember having a lovely time at a playdate. A new friend and I were chatting openly for the first time. I was hungry for connection with other mums and discussion that wasn't always baby focused.

I kept glancing over at the clock on her wall. Designated naptime was approaching. The anxiety was rising in my chest, and whilst I was really getting a lot out of our conversation, I was feeling 'itchy'. Do you get that feeling? Where you start to get restless and a part of you wants to make your excuses and do a runner. However, the sensible part of you knows you'd appear rude.

When the things we use to ground ourselves are wobbly and uncertain, it won't offer the solid ground we need.

My anxiety was getting in the way of our conversation as I was more focused on the time than what my friend was saying. I felt envious of those who could go with the flow but, at the same time, Oscar seemed to thrive in the routine we had set. Anyway, we wrapped up the conversation and Oscar went down for his nap twenty minutes late. He was tired, but it was fine.

An extra ten or twenty minutes here and there wouldn't have been the be all and end all in the grand scheme of routine, and may have offered me more opportunities to connect, linger and relax. When the things we use to ground ourselves are wobbly and uncertain, it won't offer the solid ground we need.

When you recognise that your anxiety is triggered, try to speak kindly to yourself. Anxiety is fear in action. I'm not saying throw the routine out of the window, take it on a case by case basis. Question whether your routine could be a tad more relaxed in certain instances or ordered slightly differently to accommodate your circumstances. As you gently nudge the parameters of your comfort zone, you'll grow in confidence in your newfound space.

You really feel empathy

Empathy means that you respond emotionally to others and are sensitive to their needs and feelings. Perhaps you are one of the first to recognise when another mum doesn't seem herself. You may historically be one of the people they choose to speak to when they are struggling because they feel heard, understood and warmly received. You're the one who offers a listening ear and a hot drink. And when people share their stories with you, it's like you sometimes feel a bit of what they're experiencing. You might find yourself tearful when someone else cries because you really feel for them. The stories of others impact you and stay with you for a while.

Empathy is a valuable quality. We can feel a strong sense of purpose in helping others. That is certainly not a bad thing. However, feeling a sense of purpose and believing that helping others is what makes you worthwhile are two different things. The challenge comes when our understanding of what we are worth is tied up in what we do. Other people coming to us to help them feel better can evolve into us needing to help other people in order to feel useful. We need to feel needed in order to feel worth something.

I've always been the agony aunt to everyone. It's what they call me. I feel bad when I can't answer a phone call or they want to meet. It's harder to fit stuff in now. I feel like a crap friend.

Bernie

Empathy can develop into a desire to make others happy, to please them. I lived for others for so much of my life. I call myself a people-pleaser in recovery, and it's probably a huge factor in my desire to become a therapist. Helping others gave me purpose. I felt horrendous if for any reason I'd upset or disappointed anyone. Often the guilt that I may have upset someone plagued my sleep.

Wanting to please others gives us a moral compass and makes us aware of the repercussions of our actions. However, allowing yourself to consider what is pleasing to others is different to being completely ruled by it. And I was ruled by it.

In early motherhood, not only are our personal resources (time and energy) challenged but we often are exposed to a whole new social group to please. I recall shifting and changing my personal opinions on feeding, weaning and other parenting debates depending on the attitudes of those around me.

I feared that if I expressed an opinion that was different to theirs, they'd feel offended. I wanted them to feel like I was affirming and encouraging them instead. I also remember taking it upon myself to help every new friend of mine who felt stuck, alone, down or confused. I helped people, that's what I did. That's why people liked me, right? That's why they wanted to be my friend. I was afraid that veering from always trying to please and appease people would cost me my support network.

I found myself being all, 'Yeah — baby-led weaning' because they seemed so keen. Then I'd hide the pouches when they came for coffee.

Jules

People-pleasing is addictive because no amount of thank-yous or compliments will ever satisfy a people-pleasing hunger. They provide momentary satisfaction. That's because we're using the measure of what others think about us to dictate our worth. It's not the correct currency. It's like trying to measure temperature with a ruler.

There is no fixed formula for pleasing everyone. You might bake one person a cake and they're delighted. Then you bake for someone else and discover that they're highly offended because you neglected to remember that they disliked cake. What may please one person may displease another. You simply can't please everyone all the time. No, you can't please everyone *any* of the time.

In the process of attempting to please others, we can silence our wants, needs and opinions. Each time we do this, we are telling ourselves that our feelings, opinions and needs are of less worth than someone else's. The irony is that we are trying to keep others happy in order to feel like we have more worth. Yet the reality is that we are negatively impacting our self-worth.

I spent six months trying to help my friend whose marriage was in trouble. I spoke to her most days. I spent so much time helping her that I ended up spending less time with my partner and we felt distant then too.

Krystal

A huge part of working through this people-pleasing drive is to recognise how detrimental it's been for you and how it has fuelled anxiety and fear. Once we identify this, we can begin to rationalise some of the related thoughts using grounding and coping mechanisms, and work on our self-esteem.

Bringing balance into empathy

One of my top tips for people-pleasing is to pause. For example, we invited friends to stay with us for the weekend. Amidst the morning chaos, my friend offered to read to Florence whilst I grabbed a shower. The people-pleaser in me wanted to graciously reject her offer out of fear of being a burden. I paused, thinking, it would be nice to shower without her rolling around, bored on the bathmat, and Florence really enjoys their attention.

So, I said yes. And it was nice for them and nice for me. What's more, my friend didn't turn around and say, 'Anna, that was such a sacrifice. Now you owe me.' She didn't give me the impression she felt it either. Taking small risks of deviating from our self-denying, people-pleasing behaviour builds confidence. It reinforces the fact that your needs, feelings and opinions have as much value as anyone else's.

Next time you have an opportunity to express something that you might usually swallow down, pause and consider what it might be like to share it. Next time you're asked to do something, pause and consider whether you have the extra resources to spend at present, and what it might be like to warmly decline without an extravagant flurry of apologies.

Conclusion

It's a big step to address our personality traits because these behaviours and habits have served important purposes in the past. They have enabled us to navigate and make sense of challenging situations. However, rigid personality traits exacerbate our anxiety because life and other people constantly challenge them. It can add to that sense of feeling out of control of what is happening and what others think. For example, if I need to feel like everyone is pleased with me, I feel destabilised and anxious when I am aware I have unintentionally annoyed someone.

Needing to live at either end of any personality trait spectrum in order to feel safe and grounded has drawbacks. Life is lived in all the grey areas in between. Consider the pendulum of a big antique grandfather clock. It spends a mere split second at either pinnacle of its swing, spending much more time lolling between those two points. And if it were to run out of momentum, it would settle exactly in between.

As we challenge the black and white behaviours at either ends of the spectrum, we can slowly coach ourselves towards the grey, middle ground. Try imagining a kind, inner voice coaching that fearful part of you through the little risks of authenticity you take. Kindness is important because this isn't about 'fault' or being 'wrong', it's about addressing behaviours that are holding us back from being ourselves, and feeding our anxiety.

Top Tip

Imagine a kind, inner voice coaching that fearful
part of you.

JOURNAL POINTS

- Which of these personality traits do you
  recognise in yourself?
- What are the positives and negatives of this
  trait for you?
- How would you like to address it?
- What small risks of authenticity might you take
  to bring yourself into the grey area of that trait?
- Over the next few days, note down the small
  risks you've taken and how it felt. Consider
  how those around you responded and how it
  impacted your confidence.

Chapter 8

Dismantling intrusive thoughts

Mantra: *I am not my thoughts.*

Intrusive thoughts are common, anxiety-based thoughts in which we imagine a future that has not yet happened and may not happen. They range from the humorous, like when I imagine pushing over a stand of mugs in a crowded gift shop, to the deeply disturbing. Some intrusive thoughts can be reflective of your fears or your previous experiences. However, some may directly oppose your personal beliefs and morals.

The intrusive thoughts that bother us most tend to be the darker ones that are unpleasant, scary or traumatic. They are often concealed by shame and can have so much control over our minds, actions and decisions. However, they don't need to. I am going to offer some insight into the workings and causes of intrusive thoughts. Understanding what they are and how you can address them can bring so much light into those dark places.

Intrusive thoughts needn't be a dirty secret

So many clients enter my consulting room carrying what they believe to be a shame-filled, dirty secret. They tell me, 'I have these awful thoughts and images that come into my head and make me question my sanity.' Their intrusive thoughts cause them to feel mad, terrible and alone. There is often a visible sense of relief that crosses their faces when I don't jump back in sheer horror or grab the phone to report them to the authorities.

I recently conducted an Instagram poll, asking people whether they experienced intrusive thoughts. Out of 4,500 respondents, an overwhelming 96 per cent said yes. Intrusive thoughts appear to be a universal symptom of anxiety and post-trauma, yet they go undiscussed.

It might be that you experienced intrusive thoughts before becoming a mother but perhaps they didn't seem that traumatic or shocking, or you had the energy to rationalise them. This rationality is harder to access when we are feeling tired, hormonal, stressed or depleted, which is why many mums experience an increase in intrusive thoughts during the early stages of motherhood. What's more, suddenly we feel wholly responsible for this tiny being that we love so much.

When we become mothers, we switch to a new level of alertness to risk and a whole realm of possibility and anxiety triggers. There are the rashes, SIDS risks, the fear of choking on solids or abduction. We get handed leaflets detailing the symptoms of deadly diseases that we may not previously have given a second thought to.

When I became a mother, things on TV suddenly developed an entire new level of meaning for me. I relate so much more to any news feature or storyline involving a child. My mother heart gets tightly wrung like a dishcloth. Experiencing this new level of empathy when you become a mother is understandable, but you may find that things that never used to bother you can begin to trigger anxiety and fuel intrusive thoughts.

When we become mothers, we switch to a new level of alertness to risk.

My experience with intrusive thoughts

I thought it might be helpful for me to talk you through my experience of intrusive thoughts so that you can see some of the forms they take.

I'd experienced intrusive thoughts before becoming a mother. There was a time in my life when I felt very low and depressed. My stream of thought would be harshly interrupted by visions of jumping in front of a passing car, or similar. I could mostly rationalise these because they didn't contradict my depressed state. The thoughts somehow seemed to fit within the context of how I felt.

Anyway, a few years later I had a new baby. I loved him with my whole heart. So much so that sometimes it almost hurt my eyes to look at him for too long. I walked down the creaky stairs one morning after a rough night and, BAM. I had this clear flash of him tumbling out of my arms and down the stairs.

It made me feel sick. I held him tighter, tensed my shoulders and continued downstairs at the pace of an elderly woman.

If I let my mind ruminate on these thoughts, I'd feel a heavy ache of fear, shock and grief as I played out the scenario in my mind. If you had watched me during the moments in which I envisaged the buggy rolling into a busy road, you'd have simply seen me inhaling sharply and continuing on.

Move on to postpartum period number two – Charlie was my silent reflux baby. Our days often began at midnight as he screamed around the clock. Some days I functioned (barely) on a paltry forty-five minutes of sleep. My eyes were gritty and dry, I slurred my speech and couldn't trust myself behind the wheel. It was hard to gather myself together to be consistent for Oscar. I remember how sore my skin felt due to the constant drying of my eyes on the tea towel. I wanted to hide at least some of my tears from him. I'd try to make my voice sound even. I knew he looked to me for safety and security but my words wobbled around the edges.

In my darkest, most desperate moments, I fantasised about something happening to me so that I'd be hospitalised, which would give me a break. I could sleep there. Someone would look after me. It feels shocking to see it in black and white. But I doubt that I'm alone. And if you've ever thought that and been shocked at yourself too, then there we go . . . you aren't alone.

With this low point came a different kind of intrusive thought. As I type this, I feel a wave of shame and trepidation. Will you judge me? Will you wonder what kind of mother I am? Perhaps you might consider picking up the phone to the police or a doctor, or to social services. Maybe you'd tell them they need to take my kids away.

These feelings of shame and fear keep us stuck and isolated with intrusive thoughts. They stop us from seeking supportive and grounding voices and input. During those days I struggled to see a way out. My intrusive thoughts became darker. I'd get uninvited images of me, not just dropping my dark-haired babe down the stairs, but throwing him.

My exhausted brain was desperate for relief, for respite. I struggled to complete coherent sentences, let alone process dark thoughts. Historically, I'd feel horrified at why on earth someone could shake a baby. I didn't understand. But, in my darkest times, in the darkest nights, I could empathise with the intense despair and distress those mothers must have experienced. In my situation, these thoughts weren't born out of madness; they came out of hormone-fuelled, sleep-deprived desperation. They came somewhere from a deep carnal drive for survival.

Let me reassure you – actually acting on these kinds of thoughts is incredibly rare. Speak with your health visitor, midwife or doctor. They are there to help you through this. Their aim is to put things in place to support you in your mothering, not separate you from your baby.

I went to my GP after meeting my friends for coffee for my thirty-first birthday. My friends were greatly relieved as they had been gently encouraging me to seek some support for a while. They whisked Oscar off to the park so that I could walk to the surgery with Charlie nestled in the carrier. As the doctor asked me whether I felt like I was bonding with my baby, I broke down.

On asking for support, the systems that were available to support me could be accessed and things set in motion. Friends and family who had been waiting in the wings for me to stop powering on alone felt relief at my deconstruction of the steel wall I'd built around myself. I needed people.

Now, some of my situations may sound rather extreme to some of you but will resound with others. However, that was the reality of my depths and how intrusive thoughts played a part. But it is also a story of hope and confirmation of how vulnerability is the turning point of mental health journeys. We power on because we believe that's what being a good mother is. We power on because we worry about the judgement of others. But for me, powering on in my own strength just took me deeper into my own darkness. Waving that white flag of surrender was the bravest, strongest thing I've ever done. It wasn't the end but the beginning of a better path; a path on which I wasn't alone.

These days my intrusive thoughts ebb and flow along with hormone peaks and a rough night's sleep. Seeing the patterns and the links between my physical state and the fluctuations in intrusive thoughts has been so important for me. I can rationalise them a lot more efficiently when I can put them down to the fact that I'm tired or my period is due.

I still get intrusive thoughts. I know I probably always will to varying extents. They are often focused on people I love getting sick or dying, me falling down the stairs whilst holding a child or crashing the car on the motorway. However, they don't impact my mood, actions or state of mind in the way they used to. I see them for what they are. They are cruel visions that skip across my mind. They are not certainties of my future. I've stopped feeding them their favourite form of nourishment – my attention. These days they rarely grow unless I respond to them with undeserved headspace.

Why do we get intrusive thoughts?

Our minds are creative and clever. We are constantly assessing risks, choices and possibilities as we go about our lives. Our brain considers impulses, needs, fears and desires in a single fleeting second that often goes unnoticed.

This process enables us to act and react to risk and threat quickly. As my kids scoot around our local area, my mind is calculating risk and listening for the noise of vehicles without me even realising I'm doing it. I can continue to have a coherent conversation with a friend as we walk along and then I may interrupt a sentence to shout a warning seemingly out of nowhere.

Sometimes, during periods of anxiety or increased intrusive thoughts, we can become hyper-aware of this internal process that usually bumbles along in the background. We're much more likely to hone in on obscure thoughts and consider them further if they evoke emotion such as humour, shock, fear or grief.

Instead of simply hearing the hum of an engine and checking the boys' positioning on the pavement, I might imagine a car whipping around the corner and hitting one of my boys off their scooter. Thoughts become potential scenarios as we add flesh to their bones with our imagination.

It's like we are bringing something into full colour theatre, when it was only intended to be a black and white static image.

When I do add colour to these fleeting thoughts, when I play them out as a mini film in my mind, it has a big impact on my emotions. I'm feeling shock, horror, helplessness and grief. And it feels so real. Like it's actually happening.

The challenge is that these intrusive thoughts aren't irrational. You can't easily beat them off as impossible and reassure yourself that they are never going to come to fruition. I'm conjuring up real-life, potential scenarios. These are things that do happen or have happened to me. These are things that nobody can promise will never happen.

Promising me that nothing bad will ever happen to my baby might make me feel better. However, we'd both know it would be an empty promise. Sometimes, I really want to hear it. I want my mum to walk into the room, give me a hug and promise me that my family and I will forever be safe. We are sometimes sharply aware that none of us, however careful, are immune from life's curveballs. Addressing anxiety and intrusive thoughts is a process of coming to terms with the fact that bad things happen, and seeking ways to feel peaceful amidst that truth.

What should you do about intrusive thoughts? Consider what might be fuelling them. This insight can give you strength and ground you. Insight can act like a boat anchor in the storm. The waves will still come and go, and the boat bobs with the tide, but it's safe.

Physical and mental states

The way our bodies are functioning at any one moment has an impact on our thoughts. Many of us can identify with PMT or PMS but if you struggle with anxious or intrusive thoughts, your hormonal cycles may bring an uplift in those too. I find it so helpful to connect the dots with that.

When we're compromised in any way we can find it harder to rationalise intrusive thoughts. When we're tired, unwell, hormonal, stressed or processing trauma, the thoughts can quickly gain traction so we need to utilise additional coping mechanisms to support us.

When I stopped breastfeeding, I suddenly got all these awful thoughts. Mostly about my husband dying or having an affair. So, I went to my doctor and she basically told me that my hormones were changing because I'd stopped breastfeeding. I never made the link. It was really helpful, and sure enough, the thoughts stopped coming so fast.

Iona

Trauma's part in intrusive thoughts

Like with any unwanted thoughts or behaviours, there's an extent to which they can be understood and dismantled, and life can continue. The best way to address intrusive thoughts isn't by trying to stop them as such but to address the way we interact with them.

When your intrusive thoughts carry a theme relating to

something traumatic that has happened to you, it's important to seek therapeutic support. For example, my sister's cancer diagnosis was traumatic. This explains why many of my intrusive thoughts are around my children also getting cancer. The more I have given acknowledgement to the original trauma and have allowed myself to process the resulting grief, the less pertinent and traumatising those intrusive thoughts become.

Trauma fuels anxious and intrusive thoughts. This is because the memories of our experiences can still feel present and raw. It is usually the things we've swept under the carpet that find their voice through the means of intrusive thoughts. The thing is, when we sweep them under the carpet, they aren't gone. It makes the carpet lumpy and awkward and we trip over it.

When Kian was two months old, he had to have surgery on his heart. It was terrifying but we just got through it. Then I had Ivan and it all just kept coming back to me. I'd assume he'd have issues too and I'd just keep getting these thoughts that he was going to die. I got referred for therapy for PTSD and it really helped me see how much Kian's surgery had impacted me. Sorting through that helped the thoughts I was getting.

Faye

Trauma therapy aims to help you process what you've been through. Ideally, the traumatic experience can then become a memory to be recalled at your will and less likely to be something that repeatedly forces itself on you.

How do I know if my thoughts are trauma-based or not?

Perhaps you've been shaken by these thoughts but able to carry on regardless. Maybe now, knowing that so many people experience them helps take the sting out of them. However, it's good to ask yourself whether these thoughts are affecting your daily life, decision-making confidence, relationships and behaviour.

1. They are causing you emotional distress or are traumatic in themselves.

I couldn't stop thinking of this one awful scene involving my baby. It would hit me randomly every day, multiple times. I really feared it but the more I tried to stop it, the more it came. I got therapy and we unpicked why it was happening. It's so much better. It's not like it never comes, it does sometimes but I know what it is now and I don't give it much notice.

Anonymous

2. You feel unable to control them or utilise ways to address them.

I'd lie in bed terrified that my baby would stop breathing. I'd think about the whole situation. My brain was like a runaway train and I'd end up having a panic attack pretty much every night. My husband said I needed to get some help. Fortunately,

I've got some good tools now and can tell how when I'm tired, I'm more vulnerable.

Lauren

3. You feel compelled to engage in impulsive behaviour as an attempt to control them.

I was so terrified of Tom getting meningitis after reading an article on it that I checked him all over for rashes at least three times a day. I'd strip him down naked to make sure I checked him over completely. He hated it. I felt so guilty but I couldn't stop.

Lana

4. The intrusive thoughts impact your behaviour and the decisions you make.

I literally can't believe I'm writing this but it shows how far I've come. I used to be terrified that Caleb would be abducted. I used to spiral into these thoughts and imagine it all. I wouldn't let anyone look after him that wasn't direct family, not even so I could go to the toilet. And when I took him outside, I only ever used the carrier, because I was scared someone would take the buggy. I kind of thought that the thoughts were like premonitions of what was going to happen. It's the only way I could make sense of why I had them all the time.

Fenella

My three top tips for addressing intrusive thoughts

These are my go-to techniques when I have an intrusive thought. I use them often and they can be used with all types of anxious and intrusive thoughts that barge into your brain.

1. Starve them of attention

Intrusive thoughts hunger for and grow on one kind of simple food. Their food of choice is your undivided attention.

I once had a fern. I bought it from the local garden centre. The label warned me that it was a rather high-needs plant. It had a specific list of caretaking instructions on the plastic stick I lost in the car on the way home. All I cared about was its delicate ferny leaves, looking so green and healthy on my hallway table.

I tell you, bringing that fern home was like bringing home another newborn from the hospital. It barely lasted all of a week in its happy state. As soon as it didn't have what felt like my full attention, it would quickly wilt. Needless to say, it ended up abandoned on the patio, now a crisp, sunburnt echo of its former self. I replaced it with a fake one.

Intrusive thoughts will come, regardless of what you do. But you have a choice in how or whether you interact with them.

Intrusive thoughts will come. But as we focus on them, we water them. We nurture them. They grow bigger and stronger and more controlling very quickly. By indulging them with our attention, we are inviting them to take space in our mind that, frankly, they don't deserve. As we apply less meaning to their content, we can grow in confidence that they are thoughts, not premonitions or future certainties.

2. Imagine the boring, mundane alternative

I've been using this technique a lot lately and I'm finding it helpful. Every time I get an intrusive or anxious thought, I encourage myself to think of the boring, mundane alternative.

Say for example that Florence has a temperature at bedtime. It's not unexpected as the boys have recently passed a cold between themselves. She has no further symptoms that I feel worried about. I suddenly get an intrusive thought that her temperature is caused by something sinister.

The temptation may then be to pick up my phone and go on an internet-searching rampage. My anxiety would increase second by second as I'd find myself frantically scrolling through forums, skim-reading harrowing stories. I'd be on high alert, adrenaline-filled and waiting for the next telling symptom to appear and confirm my fears. Maybe I'd then sleep restlessly, struggling to ground myself in the simple facts of the matter.

In this situation I could use the technique of imagining the mundane, more likely alternative. I'd counteract my intrusive thought of horrendous illness by imagining her waking up with a bit of a snotty nose and a temperature that paracetamol could address.

If you find this technique helpful, you can use this for all types of anxiety. For example, social anxiety: 'everyone at this party thinks I'm boring' can be counteracted with, 'nobody is thinking anything about me at all because they are focusing on having a nice time'. Even if you don't find yourself falling for the mundane alternative every time, it's good to conjure it up, as it's often far more realistic and statistically probable.

Should our initial fears or concerns happen, we will react and address them at that time, rather than living through them in our minds regardless. Playing out scenarios in our mind is emotionally draining. It is more beneficial to preserve that emotional energy for situations as they arise, rather than spend it on situations that may never come to pass.

3. Mop man

I like to talk about a mop salesman. I've no idea where I got this analogy – somewhere in the deep and creative places of my mind – but this technique is for you if you enjoy some imagery.

Imagine that you are sitting down with your dinner on a Friday night. It's 8 p.m. The baby is finally sound asleep and you're shattered. You put a film on, grab a tray of comfort food and exhale as you flop onto the sofa. You've been looking forward to this moment all day.

And then, suddenly, the doorbell rings. You launch out of your seat in case they dare ring again and wake the baby. Who on earth is ringing your doorbell at this time of the evening?

You open the door to find a man selling mops – 'I'd like

to introduce you to my new range of mega mops. Clean your floor in half the time,' he says, grinning expectantly. Whilst the tiles you're standing on could undoubtedly do with a thorough clean, you don't need a mop. You need to be knee-deep in comfort food and episode four of your boxset.

You feign interest. 'Come on in,' you say. In he walks, mops clattering against the doorframe. Before you know it, he's sitting on your sofa with his shoes off, talking passionately about the Supersplash G76 and sipping on the glass of wine you've offered him out of politeness. 'Want some chips, we've got plenty?' you say. He gladly accepts as if he'd been waiting for you to ask. You eye up the clock, wondering quite how you ended up in this situation. If he makes himself at home any further, you're going to have to introduce him to your baby as 'uncle'. You feel invaded.

What could an alternative scenario be? The doorbell rings, you answer it hastily. 'I'd like to introduce you to my new range of mega mops. Clean your floor in half the time.' You smile back and say, 'I'm all good for mops but thanks for stopping by.' Off he goes to wake next door's kids. You close the door and resume your film.

Intrusive thoughts, they will come. We can feel intruded upon by them and passive to them, but we do have a choice:

1. Invite the thoughts in and focus on them. Use your active, creative imagination to turn the black and white thought into an elaborate full-colour story. This leaves you feeling anxious, exhausted and confused. Your brain registers a threat so your sympathetic nervous system kicks in and things could spiral into panic.

2.   Recognise that you are not passive to intrusive thoughts. You cannot control how often they come and what they are but you can control how much authority you give them through attention. Wave the thought on by.

Intrusive thoughts are not reflective of your personality

These are a few of my go-to techniques that might help you. Distraction and grounding techniques also aid you in reclaiming control.

If you have cruel thoughts that hop into your mind like an unwelcome visitor when you're simply getting on with life, remember that they do not reflect your personality. The thought might seem crazy but *you* are not. It's not the thought itself that is a problem; it's what you do with it.

Intrusive thoughts *are* not reflective of your personality.

Be kind and patient with yourself as you address intrusive thoughts. Your mind is used to responding to them in a certain way, and therefore challenging and changing that can take time. Even if you manage to halt one spiral out of five, that is a victory. We're equipping and retraining our brains to react differently.

I know I've touched on this before but if intrusive thoughts are causing you distress, please seek support like I did. You are worth finding the tools to live your life without being bombarded by traumatic thoughts. Intrusive thoughts don't deserve a position of dominance where they rob your motherhood experience of all enjoyment and peace.

Top Tip

Next time you get a horrible intrusive thought, encourage yourself to think of the boring, mundane alternative.

JOURNAL POINTS

- Do you identify with having intrusive thoughts?
- How does it feel to have this extra understanding of what they are?
- Do your intrusive thoughts have particular themes? What are they?
- Might you have experienced any trauma that could be fuelling them? If so, consider seeking support to help process it.
- Have you noticed what increases or decreases the amount of intrusive thoughts you experience?
- Which of these techniques might you like to try?

Chapter 9

Talking about your internal dialogue

Mantra: *I deserve the compassion I give my child.*

How often do you find yourself overthinking the words you've spoken or the ones uttered to you? You are also aware of how the tone of voice and the words spoken to your child impact how loved and safe they feel. Words can create community and connection. They encourage, inspire, support. But they can also deconstruct, discourage, destroy.

However, the most significant conversation you'll ever have takes place in the secret depths of your mind. It's the foundation to your inner world. It informs the way you interact with others, your level of self-worth and the decisions you make. Your internal dialogue might blend into the background but it has the potential to be the

Your internal dialogue might blend into the background but it has the potential to be the biggest threat to your sense of self.

biggest threat to your sense of self. We're going to shine a light on it and see how your internal dialogue can become your biggest supporter as you work on your anxiety.

The character of your internal dialogue

First, let's consider the characteristics of your internal voice. For most of my life, my inner dialogue was unforgiving, strict, perfectionist and critical. This is incredibly common in anxiety so I wouldn't be surprised if yours carried a similar tone. The thing is, we don't see how much of our lives that this type of constant dialogue affects until we really start to notice it. And that's what I want to draw to your attention in this chapter.

Speaking to ourselves in this way has the same effect on us as if we'd had an angry teacher standing over our work relentlessly criticising every mark we made. Over the years, it crushes our sense of self-esteem and chip, chip, chips away at our sense of self-worth.

Can you imagine speaking to your baby, a friend or loved one in the way you speak to yourself? Consider the impact it would have on their sense of worth. Wouldn't it shape their understanding of who they are? It would impact whether they believe they are loveable, or enough.

So how does this relate to motherhood? It relates in every way. It affects how understanding and patient of ourselves we are as we get our heads round this new role. It's harder to make the faltering steps of any transition in life when we have this voice inside our heads telling us that we aren't doing good enough, learning fast enough, getting enough done.

This cruel inner self-chat inflames mum-guilt like fuel thrown on a small flicker of fire. Who needs constant criticism when they're trying to navigate a life that looks totally different to how it did a few months ago?

Cruel inner self-chat fuels mum guilt.

Would you criticise and berate an intern for not functioning like the CEO?

In my head, I was always telling myself that I wasn't good enough for Evan. I always felt I was failing him. The guilt was constant.

Abi

My internal dialogue

I will forever be working on my internal dialogue. It's like the eternal restoration of a big old, tumbledown property. You know the ones? The ones my parents used to take great delight in dragging us round. The ones that now we buy yearly membership to enable us to visit whenever we fancy. (There's a high chance I'm turning into my mum. Fortunately, that's not a bad thing.)

In these big old buildings, people work around the clock to restore the sun-bleached artwork and weathered stone. They dust, varnish, paint and sand. There is always work to be done. As old wear and tear is attended to, new bumps and scrapes are created. Just as staff maintain the detail of these buildings, I need to conduct regular maintenance on my internal dialogue. We all do.

After having Charlie and feeling so low, I realised quite

how cruel my internal dialogue had become. It had gone unchecked and unmaintained for a long time. It had land-slid so far in fact that I felt like an utter failure as a mother. I wouldn't be told otherwise. I saw my unsettled, unhappy baby and felt him to be concrete proof of my failure. To counteract this, I applied all the energy I had available into concealing my shameful failure from the world. I must appear to have it together.

I turned down practical and emotional support when offered. It felt vulnerable to think that people had seen through my cracking veneer. As a result, my defences would fly up like an impenetrable shield. 'I'm fine,' I'd squeak. I wasn't. So relentlessly critical and unkind was my inter-nal dialogue, I fundamentally believed I was a failure if I accepted support that I wasn't worthy of anyway.

On hitting a rather messy rock bottom, I became aware of how cruel my internal dialogue had become. I started to slowly address it and those rusty cogs began to grind to a squeaky halt and slowly clunk, and creak into a healthier, kinder and more compassionate reverse.

I'm still working on it and, realistically, probably always will be. I need to, for the sake of my internal and external life. Don't I notice when I take my foot off the gas and try to freewheel a while. I feel like working on my internal dialogue is a constant undoing. It's an undoing and an unpicking of all that the world tries to tell us about ourselves.

You are OK.

You are enough.

The most worthwhile investment

I sure make addressing your internal dialogue sound like a lot of hard work. But let me tell you something (if you take one thing from this chapter, let it be this) – addressing your internal dialogue and introducing a kinder voice, is possibly *the* worthiest investment of your time and energy. Ever. There is not one thing in my life, one tiny dark nook that has gone untouched by the fact that I have challenged my internal dialogue. Going up a downward escalator it may indeed feel like at times, but I'll continue the plod because the quality of my life and relationships depend on it.

Your inner conversation is the most significant conversation you'll ever have.

Addressing my internal dialogue has shifted my sense of worth. This has in turn changed where I place my boundaries with people. It has attended to my belief that everyone else's needs were worthier than mine. It has shifted my belief that I'm only valuable for what I can do, give to, help with and be for others. It has changed my standards on how I'm treated. It has made me slowly realise I'm worthy of the love I am given from my husband, my family, my kids. It has given me the ability to seek and accept support and help. It has given me a voice and the increasing confidence to use it. It has chipped away at perfectionism and is replacing it with 'enough is enough'. I apologise less for taking up space in the world. The acrid whisper of 'yeah, but if you really knew me ...' has softened and quietened. I'm a work in progress. I will always be a work in progress. Yes, it is work.

But goodness me, it is good to feel, live and love in the mess of the progress.

Let's do this.

But I don't think I have an inner dialogue . . .

I don't even think I have an inner voice. All I hear is my thoughts.
                                                              Rudy

We all have an inner commentary. It might have gone unnoticed and unchallenged for so long that it has become wallpaper to you. It might not be an audible voice. It might be a stream of quiet thoughts or feelings that run like a thread through your mind.

Start to pay attention to what your mind says. It's more likely to be noticeable when your emotions or stress levels peak or something unexpected happens. You might notice it pop up when you drop the bottle of painfully expressed milk or fear you're losing your grip during the tenth wake-up of the night. It's in moments like this where we can start to identify what this dialogue sounds like. Mine used to be, 'Oh you idiot, you stupid girl.'

It's a case of starting to consciously listen out for it. As you do, you'll notice it more as time goes on. You'll become more sensitive to the tone and the language. And *then* you'll be in a good position to address it.

How the inner dialogue is shaped

Consider how your inner dialogue has been shaped. This dialogue begins at an early age and gains momentum as we grow. We build our internal voice out of our experience of the way people speak to us and treat us.

If your parents or caregivers were kind and loving, patient and reassuring, that's a great start. This is always the ideal scenario and what we all hope to offer our children.

But life is often more complex than that, and not all of us have been lucky enough to be brought up in this way. When there has been verbal abuse, criticism or bullying throughout our lives, then the work can be a bit more challenging. It might be that you remember a particularly cruel teacher or a harsh relative. It's also tricky when those influencing us aren't speaking kindly of themselves as we can absorb this cruel dialogue even if it's not directed at us.

My mum was always accepting but my dad, he wanted a lot for me. He wanted me to achieve a lot at school. It came from wanting the best but I always felt pressured and feared letting him down. I guess that might be where my perfectionism came from. I don't want Toby to grow up feeling this way so I'm trying to be more relaxed about my expectations, for both of us.

Tania

Whether an event or the words of others informed your internal language, it does not mean it's true. People speak out of their own brokenness; however, you don't have to live your life with a hurtful dialogue echoing through your actions and relationships like the words etched through a stick of seaside rock.

Harsh inner dialogues can get passed down through generations, impacting each generation somehow. Sometimes you can see these traits. You might see how your father and your grandfather both have very high perfectionist traits and get their sense of worth from highly achieving and feeling deep shame when they miss their own, self-set mark.

Perhaps you also see this trait in yourself and you've felt the weight of it on your shoulders throughout your schooling and career. You feel like you really want to encourage your son or daughter to have more realistic and kinder expectations of their own achievements. Perhaps you felt like you had to do well to please your father, and experienced a sense of failure when you didn't get the grades he hoped you would. You want your child to feel equally loved regardless of the grade penned on their homework.

If that's the case, it can end with you. When we address our internal dialogues, we begin to see ourselves differently and we end up parenting differently. I see the work I do on my mental health as a gift to my children. I'm doing it for me; I'm doing it for them. It's not selfish or self-absorbed to invest in caring for your mental health, it's courageous. I see it as a way of loving those who love you.

Your ability to feel loved

As I speak more kindly to myself in my mind, I act more kindly to myself. My children see that I deem myself worthy of respect and care. Therefore, it encourages them to believe that they and others must also be worthy of respect and care.

The thing is, we can only accept and allow love from others to the extent that we love ourselves. Honestly. I'll explain – say you could give your value as a number out of ten. There have been significant times in my life where I felt I was worth two out of ten. Almost worthless, but not completely, because I did nice things for people and that made me worth something. I used to say to my own mother, 'You have to say you love me because you're my mum.' And of my friends I used to feel that they only liked me because they didn't *really* know me. I felt like an imposter in pretty much every relationship I had.

And then my now husband came along. Our eyes met across a crowded, sticky bar. He was good to me, kind to me. He liked me. He thought I was worth far more than the two out of ten value I placed on myself. He thought I was ten out of ten.

Part of me couldn't believe my luck. A larger part of me found this incredibly uncomfortable. I was holding my breath, waiting for him to discover that I was actually quite rubbish and nowhere near as worthy of his time, attention and affection as he believed. Sometimes, I'd try to prove it by attempting to sabotage our relationship or break up with him. His anger would have felt more comfortable than his love. I'm still pretty surprised we made it through those years.

As my internal dialogue has changed and become kinder, my self-worth has changed. Whilst I have my moments when my resilience is low and my internal dialogue has gone unchecked for a while, I do believe I am loveable. The love from my friends, family and children is easier to receive.

If you place your worth at two out of ten and someone comes along and tells you that you're worth ten out of ten, you're going to find it hard to accept and to receive the attention and affection that they think you're worth. I tell you what; your child is going to grow up to think the world of you. And that will be so much easier to receive if you have grown to believe that ultimately you are loveable, as they are.

You'll get things wrong sometimes. Maybe a lot of times. Things may be messy some days, inside and outside your head. You're a glorious, complex mess of humanity. But we all are.

Do you believe your baby is less worthy of your love when they reject the food you made or had a wakeful night? No, because you don't experience their worth as a moveable entity. The same goes for you; it's the words of your internal dialogue (and maybe some unloving people along the way) that have done a good job of persuading you otherwise for so long.

But my harsh voice keeps me in check

I've spoken to many people who are cautious about addressing their internal dialogue. They credit it for their high standards, perfectionism or rigidity. These characteristics can increase the likelihood of us feeling shame and guilt but they can also get us to good places. Perhaps your perfectionist drive has enabled you to get promotions at work because you ensure everything is done to such a high standard.

> *My inner critic drives me to be the best mum I can be. Yes, it makes me feel guilty sometimes, but it also keeps my standards high. I'm scared that being kinder to myself will make me drop my standards as a mum.*
>
> Barbs

I don't believe that if we address our internal dialogue, it means that we will achieve less and do things to a lesser standard. It may be that things change as we respect our own resources and boundaries more, but, ultimately, it's a good thing. Let me explain.

Imagine jumping ahead a few years to when it's time to apply for school places. You are viewing two schools, both are local and convenient. Both get consistently brilliant results in league charts and tables.

However, the schools are different. When you visit the first school, you sense an air of fear. Your shoulders tense and you worry that you'll put a foot wrong. You discover that the school achieves their great results through harsh, strict discipline and fear. The children are reprimanded if they don't learn at the rate they are expected. Detention and nerve-wracking chats with the angry-looking headmaster are doled out liberally. Children are regularly singled out in front of the class and shamed if they do not recall their times tables fast enough or spell a complex word correctly first time.

The other school feels completely different as you walk through. You hear laughter and you see children smiling and playing happily. The teachers seem kind and manage to discipline with a firm voice that doesn't shout. The children seem to know where to go and what to do. Rules are clearly enforced and, when children misbehave, there is a discussion and an opportunity to apologise and correct their behaviour next time. The focus is on praising positive behaviour.

Which one would you rather place your child in? Remember, both schools are ranked the same and get the same results using two very different techniques. It's an obvious choice when we put it like this. So why choose the harsh voice on yourself? You could get to where you want to be with a kind, internal supporter, rather than an angry headmistress who barks orders and criticisms.

Putting your internal dialogue into perspective

Consider how your child would respond if you spoke to them with the same tone or words that you use to speak to yourself in the secrecy of your mind. What would it do to their self-esteem and sense of worth? I find that this exercise really brings the importance of addressing our internal dialogue into sharp clarity.

People are so taken aback when I ask this because it's awful to even contemplate speaking to our kids in the critical way we speak to ourselves. I cannot imagine barking 'you idiot' at my son as he fumbles with the buttons on his school polo shirt that he's wearing for the first time. Nor would I bark 'not good enough' at my daughter as she tips over onto the cushion whilst learning to sit.

The thing is, if you don't deem the kind of chatter you use in your mind good enough for your children, then it's not good enough for you either. They deserve patience, the space to make mistakes, to get it wrong, to learn. They deserve forgiveness when they act out on difficult emotions. And so do you. It sometimes helps to think of it that way, to externalise it so that we can gain valuable perspective.

Eugh. Of course, it would devastate me if I ever imagined Austin speaking to himself in the way I speak to myself. I'd be so kind to him and desperate to make him feel better about himself.

Hannah

In recognising and addressing our internal dialogues, the choices we make can begin to change. This is because the foundations on which we make them start to be different. It might be that you always say 'yes' to the things people ask of you, regardless of whether you have the personal resources to fulfil them. Perhaps by addressing your inner critic, you begin to realise that your worth isn't entirely based on giving yourself away to others, so you choose to say no to something. This enables you to preserve extra energy and time for your family.

I started to do kinder things for myself and related to people from a place of believing I was acceptable, rather than constantly feeling I needed to earn that acceptance. I am more able to say, 'hey, I need help, I'm struggling', than plod on regardless, slowly edging towards some sort of messy meltdown.

It's tough, but the toughest changes are often the most transforming. Let's look at how you can change this internal chat.

How to grow a compassionate voice

Asking you to change what might have been an unchallenged internal dialogue for years is a big ask, I know that. But if things are to really change, that harsh critic must slowly evolve into a kind, forgiving and supportive one. That might sound like night versus day to you now but I promise it is possible.

When I talk about a kind, forgiving and supportive voice, does that sound like anyone you know or have known in your life? Maybe you're thinking of an old teacher or a family member. It might be a friend or a distant relative who isn't alive anymore. It doesn't matter who it is, it matters that you can remember how it feels to be spoken to like that. To have your doubts, concerns and failings responded to in kindness.

Your harsh critic will slowly evolve into a kind, forgiving and supportive one.

Collect these nice, kind voices like a magpie collects shiny things. Just as your critical inner dialogue has been formed along the way from the words and treatment of others, you can grow your kind inner voice in the same way.

When you find your internal dialogue up to its old

tricks, ask yourself what would someone say if you spoke all these words out loud? What would one of the people you thought of say to you in response? They would hopefully use kind, compassionate, encouraging and understanding responses, so this is how you must speak back to the critical voice.

When you're practising speaking kindly to yourself, you might want to conjure up the actual voice of someone you know. If they are a warm, kind and supportive influence, it can work well.

When I notice I'm being impatient with myself, I always remember my auntie. She would always see when I was frustrated and would speak so calmly to me I try to use her voice in my mind and imagine how she'd talk to me. It really helps.

                                                                Sam

As you continue to do this, you'll get to know your internal dialogue well. You'll start to recognise it in action much quicker and you'll begin to know the patterns of when it strikes. Maybe it increases when you're tired or stressed. Be encouraged; whilst it might feel at times like you go one step forward and two steps back, there's a point where the balance tips and the grind isn't so hard.

On dropping the pan of steamed vegetables you were about to blend for your baby's dinner, your internal dialogue might say, 'You idiot. Look what you've done!'

The compassionate voice might say, 'Ooops. These things happen! Give her a breadstick whilst you clear this up and defrost something from the freezer.'

It's tough, but the toughest changes are often the most transforming.

The Monster

Here's a slightly different way to address your internal dialogue. Often, I talk through a couple of different techniques in the hope that if one doesn't resound for you, then you might find another one will. This one is for those who learn best through imagery. We're going to take that internal dialogue outside your head and see if that helps.

OK, I want you to imagine a monster on your shoulder. This monster is your cruel inner dialogue. Take it outside your mind. It doesn't belong in there because it is *not* you. Stick it on your shoulder like a miniature ugly squawking parrot. Or shove it on the floor by your foot like one of those yappy handbag dogs.

The monster's dialogue is *not* yours, its voice isn't yours either. Its squeaky sentences are formed of words and phrases you've heard from those who've hurt, bullied or abused you. Its tone is not kind, encouraging or compassionate. Imagine what your monster looks like, what it sounds like. Mine has purple and green warty skin with long hairy fingers. It is small and almost round. It boasts coarse greying, wild eyebrows that leap away from its face.

Your monster feasts hungrily on attention. It grows bigger and sweatier, uglier and louder every time you listen to it, agree with it, act on what it says.

Start choosing to ignore the monster. He's had control for

long enough now. Every time you remove your attention from him, he shrinks and his voice becomes quieter. Every time you choose to listen to that kinder, more rational voice, he shrinks. Every time you do something kind for yourself in opposition to the things he says, or every time you express a need or accept support, his voice gets even quieter.

Unfortunately, the monster will never go away. We all have them. Even the person you know with the healthiest self-esteem of all. But we can change his size and volume by starving him of his nutrition – attention, self-criticism, self-abuse and self-denial. Sometimes he will be bigger and louder but that's OK: reprioritise using your techniques and you'll soon be turning your attention elsewhere. Better it be a tiny, squeaky monster darting around the sole of your shoe, than a towering beast blocking your sunlight.

I used to call myself a failure the whole time. My dad would always make out I'd done everything wrong. That nothing I could do would be good enough. I really believed it. I turned that inner talk into his voice. As if it was him saying it to me and not me. And then I remember all of the kind stuff people have said. And all the good things I've been told I've done. And I would remember my sister and best friend's voice telling me that I was good and that they loved me the way I was. It took a while, but my dad's voice is quieter. I feel like it's even affected the way I walk. Like, I hold my head higher. I don't have to hide and apologise anymore. I don't have to fear my inner voice beating me up because I know it wasn't me all along.

Anonymous

Top Tip

When practising speaking kindly to yourself, it can help to imagine the voice of someone you know.

JOURNAL POINTS

- What characteristics does your inner voice have?
- Is the way you speak to yourself reminiscent of the way someone has spoken to you?
- How do you think your inner dialogue impacts your mental health?
- Would you speak to someone you love in the way you speak to yourself? If not, why not?
- How are you planning on bringing compassion into your internal dialogue?

Chapter 10

Self-care = self-preservation

Mantra: *Self-care cultivates self-worth.*

'Self-care' is a rather fashionable phrase these days. I've seen it mentioned so many times that I worry people are becoming numb to it. Self-care is often spoken about in terms of treating yourself well. 'Book yourself in for a manicure, do some yoga, slide into a wonderful bubbly bath.' Whilst I'm in full support of those things, self-care is far more important than doing nice things for yourself. It's about preserving your resources and keeping yourself safe. I like to think about it as self-preservation.

This chapter looks at why self-care is such an important habit to instil when tackling anxiety, but also for life too! If you've found yourself eye-rolling at the term too, give me five minutes and I'll bring you back round to it.

Self-care and self-esteem

Most people struggling with anxiety have a lower level of self-esteem and sense of self-worth. Small acts of self-care go a long way in starting to shift how we feel about ourselves. I'm not talking about massages, meditation and long autumnal walks; I'm talking about starting with meeting your basic needs of food, warmth, hydration and shelter.

> **Small acts of self-care go a long way in starting to shift how we feel about ourselves.**

Have you ever hopped around the kitchen for an hour, desperately needing a wee when the loo is so close you can even see the bathroom door from where you stand? Have you ever sat there encouraging your babe to sip the last dregs of milk, or take a sip of water and then realised you've not drunk a single full glass all day long? Perhaps you've spent five minutes coaxing flailing limbs into warm layers and then gone out shivering because you couldn't be bothered to dig out your coat.

Last winter I loaded the car up with all the kids' stuff for a day out. As I shut the house, I realised I'd forgotten my coat. I looked at my watch. We needed to go so I left it. I was so cold that day, right down to my bones. I wish I had just left ten seconds later. I'd have done so if it was for one of the kids' coats.

Phoebe

Start addressing the basics. You meet your baby's basic needs (and far more) because you believe they are worth it. So why aren't you?

My journey with self-care

For much of my life, I wouldn't say there was a whole lot of self-care going on. Throughout my childhood, I didn't believe I had much worth because the words and actions I observed often implied otherwise. As a result, treating myself as someone of value wasn't going to be instinctive. Despite having some wonderful, nurturing and loving input in my life, it's often the hurtful influences that we give more value to, isn't it?

Instead of acting from a place of self-care, I tended to act self-destructively. This manifested in many ways over the years but I struggled to tend to even my basic needs. I'd go hungry, I'd go thirsty and I'd bully myself internally and externally through my actions. My behaviour, whilst not always overt and noticeable, was often tinged with self-sabotage, self-destruction and self-denial. I would say that there have been numerous periods of my life where I've hated myself. So why on earth would I ever desire to care for myself?

In the early days of dating my husband I remember one particular moment. During a (potentially vodka and Red Bull-fuelled) deep and meaningful late-night chat, he told me of a girl he knew who had self-harmed. As a teenager, on discovering that she'd caused herself purposeful pain, he had been shocked and saddened that someone would intentionally choose to treat themselves badly.

I didn't say it to him then but that self-destructive drive was very familiar to me. However, what was more eye opening to me was the fact it seemed such an alien concept to him. Maybe, I thought, not everyone wages a war against him- or herself.

One of the very first topics of my psychotherapy master's degree was on the self-destructive drive. I learnt that the most effective ways to counteract many of our self-destructive traits was to do the opposite. Self-care is one of the greatest ways to address the inner bully, I didn't know it then but self-care was going to be my saviour. More than once and in more than one way.

Actions speak so loudly, don't they? I began to take an umbrella when it was raining, eat when I was hungry, drink when I was thirsty. I started small and carried on small. I've learnt that, slowly but surely, these little things make big differences. Each action of self-care slowly chipped away at my low self-esteem and lack of self-worth, weakening the infrastructure that had taken such deep hold over me.

Oh man, I adore my kids. And I tell them all the time. So much so that Oscar often finishes my sentence for me. I say, 'Oscar', and he follows with 'love you'. He hears it all the time but what makes him feel it is my actions: the hugs, the caretaking, the listening, the comforting. That's what makes him believe my declarations of love, that's what makes him feel loved. Words are merely air without the substance of behaviour and action.

That's what has you believing the words they say. In fact, the words become secondary. Actions speak far louder. It's the same with self-worth. You can repeat all the self-love mantras that Pinterest has to offer but they will be merely water off a duck's back without the acts of self-care to back it up.

Anyway, fast-forward a few years to my first maternity leave. I found it hard to rest. You know that strange window of time between finishing work and the baby arriving? Everything was about to change and I remember feeling like a spare part in my own home. Not being one for sitting still, I felt like I had to justify my time not working. Nobody wanted me to justify it, in fact, people told me to make the most of it. But my worth was so wrapped up in 'doing' that it struggled to just 'be'. I ran errands I didn't need to run. I created work for myself. Looking back, I wish I could have told myself to slow the heck down; to indulge in a boxset or take the mornings slowly. However, I know full well that I wouldn't have listened. Slowness felt like an indulgence that clearly, on some level, I didn't feel deserving of.

After having Oscar I had a generally lovely time navigating life with a baby. I dabbled in a few hours of client work whilst he napped at a friend's house, I juggled but not in a way that felt overwhelming. Things felt fairly well compartmentalised. There were work hours and home hours, and time for the endless admin during baby-nap windows. Life was full but not stressful.

And then I had Charlie. And things got rather messy, as you know, with the sleep deprivation and the postnatal depression. I had the desperate need to do it all myself, in order to prove to everyone that I was a wholly capable mother with zero risk of my falling apart. And then I did fall apart and it was messy.

Life had levelled up, but my care of myself hadn't followed suit. The cost of neglecting my mental health and self-care became higher. As I did less, my self-esteem dropped. And with it, my mood dropped too. The creaky gears started to roll in the opposite direction.

Rock bottom

My self-care was utterly non-existent and I didn't feel an ounce of motivation to change that. But I had to. So much depended on it. I needed the light to be switched back on in my life, for the sake of my kids and my husband. I might not have felt worth it, but they were.

If I had waited until I felt deserving of self-care before I put things into action, it wouldn't have happened. I had to do it regardless. I began fitting exercise into tiny windows of my day, ten minutes here and there to get some endorphins flowing. I began to stock my fridge with pots of soup and pitta breads to ensure I ate. I picked up the phone to tell friends I was struggling, not so they could fix me but so I didn't feel alone. I put Oscar into a lovely, local nursery two mornings a week so that I could find some time to rest and bond with Charlie.

I invited my husband (who I'd sent to the spare room at this point as I hated him seeing me in such a hopeless state during the night), to come back into our room to give me emotional support during the endless night wakings. And, importantly, I began to usher that compassionate voice back into my head, to help me fight the bully that was repeatedly calling me a failure. It had got so loud and big, I could barely hear anything else.

These things didn't feel instinctive for a good while but I knew they were important for the sake of my family. And none of them look like a spa break or a hot bath. But they are all self-care and, in time, they began to wrench the big old creaky cog of the downward spiral in the opposite direction.

Fast-forward again to Christmas 2017. I reached burnout. My social media account had grown and the juggle of a busy household alongside an increasingly demanding job that wasn't bringing in enough money to cover the day's childcare I had. Classically, something had to get edged out of my life to make space for everything else. There were many non-negotiables, so it was any form of self-care that got nudged out of the picture. It wasn't a conscious decision, it was one of those slow things that you don't realise has left until you are suddenly faced with the consequences of its absence.

Everyone was faced with the consequences of its absence. My family had to deal with irritable, snappy me. I resented my husband for the luxurious time he spent on the train, scrolling, snoozing, catching up on emails. I mean, when you start fantasising about someone's long, sweaty commute on a packed, often delayed train, or their opportunity to stand alone in the nook of a stranger's armpit on the tube, then there's something badly awry, right?

Shutting down selfishness

A couple of years ago, my husband marched me to the local gym, boasting saunas and a crèche. He signed me up there and then. It wasn't purely for my benefit. He and the kids needed me to prioritise finding some breathing space. They were not benefitting from me being my burnt-out, knackered, resentful self. And I was reminded again that self-care wasn't selfish, it's a form of loving those who love you and have to be around you.

I have to remind myself of that often. The guilt that knocks on our door when we take a step to refill and refuel isn't about selfishness, although it may feel that way whilst we find our feet, as we recognise quite how much it benefits those around us.

Now, life has stepped up a gear again. I'm currently juggling a busy household, three kids, settling Oscar into school and writing this book (plus all the usual emails and life admin). A couple of weeks ago, I felt burnout knocking at my door. That irritability, the exhaustion and the snappiness. The sense of, 'If one more person asks another single thing of me, I may cry/scream/run for the hills.'

It's a red flag when I find myself in a place where going to the loo feels like a mini holiday. It's a warning light when accepting something nice like a compliment feels uncomfortable. I saw that my internal dialogue was sounding increasingly less 'kind parent' and more 'angry teacher'. When life levels up, we need to refill more often.

As I write now, I've sat down at my desk and put Florence down for her nap. We drove twenty minutes so that I could have a read and a shower. Florence went into the crèche for an hour where she gets fought over by the team who are seduced by her smiles and curly mop. It would have been far easier to come home, do some emails, and tick some boxes. Instead I feel rested and refreshed, ready for the impending chaos of winding down the country roads to do the school and nursery pick-up.

I still remember the huge pang of guilt I felt when I did

the same with Charlie a couple of years ago. But that guilt has ebbed away now. It's funny but when I have a bath, breathe for a few minutes, open a book or listen to a podcast and I feel like I'm doing a good thing for everyone. This is a giant leap for a girl who, a few short years ago, didn't feel that she deserved to put her tired feet up on the sofa when forty weeks pregnant.

It's not just about me. It's not just about you.

Hopefully you've taken something from my own journey of self-care. It's something we always need to monitor and keep an eye on as it has such a huge impact on our well-being. It really supports the work you are starting to do on your internal dialogue. It is the actions that really help shift that critical internal voice into a more compassionate one.

Start at the beginning

It's all very well asking you to take care of yourself and start to meet some of your needs, but first we need to become more sensitive to what they might be.

> *What do I need? Honestly, I'm not even sure any more.*
>
> Gita

We are always monitoring our children's needs. It has likely become the background noise in your brain. You watch the clock to gauge when your baby might next need a nap or a feed. We watch for yawns, grumpiness, rubbed eyes . . .

If you think they're hungry, you don't say, 'Ah, you're

hungry? No problem. I'll feed you tomorrow when I'm not so busy.' When bedtime rolls around you don't declare, 'Eugh. I really can't face getting you upstairs, into pyjamas and bed. Wait until I've finished this boxset and if I'm not asleep myself, I'm on it.'

We watch for their needs, we monitor them, we are sometimes mindful of when they need something before they even realise they do. And we take steps to meet them as soon as we can. Why? Because we value them and therefore we place value on their needs. We have a responsibility to them. We know them best.

The thing is, we mums are often so preoccupied in meeting the needs of others that we've started to lose the language of our own internal voice going, 'Hey. I'm hungry. Hello, I really need to take a breather. I need the loo.'

There have been an increasing number of days recently where come 3 p.m. I feel rather odd – all lightheaded and not very present. Then I realise I've not eaten anything beyond a banana. Not intentionally. I've simply deprioritised my needs so many times that I slip out of a three-meals-a-day routine whilst ensuring everyone else in my household gets theirs. Whether you've been there, or you are there, let me tell you now. Your needs are equally as valuable and valid as your child's.

You need to start checking in on yourself like you do with your kids. When you wonder whether they're hungry, thirsty or tired, ask yourself too. Obviously, we can't indulge in sumptuous two-hour naps in the middle of the day (or maybe you can. If so, go you!). But take a moment to acknowledge your tiredness and see how you might meet that need, along with others. It might be that it helps connect the dots of why you're feeling emotional or snappy today, so that you can show yourself some empathy.

Start getting in touch with the language of your own needs again. Ask yourself, 'What do I need?' Whether it can be met in that moment, or not at all, sometimes simply being able to acknowledge it for yourself is important.

Maybe you need a holiday but you can't see that happening for another 3,782 years. Let's break it down. What is it about a holiday that you need? Some headspace? Some time to relax? A change of scenery?

I wonder what you can do for yourself that might be able to give you an ounce of that somehow. Would it be possible to pack up the car and drive to a friend's house out of town for a different environment? Or perhaps you can ask someone to watch your baby for an hour whilst you escape into a book and have a long shower. It's not the same as a week on a pool lounger but it's certainly something. You might crave dinner with a friend but your baby is going through a growth spurt. Perhaps it's connection and conversation you're craving. If the meal isn't possible, schedule a phone call and chat whilst you walk the baby in the buggy.

> *Sometimes I just feel like I need some space but my partner works away. I ended up having to pay someone to come for a couple of hours a week but it actually made all the difference.*
>
> Su

Regardless of whether your need can be met or not, acknowledge it if you can, because it is still valid. You may need to hear the comforting words of a family member who has passed away, or you may wish for older, simpler days. Sometimes there's a sense of loss, resentment, grief, sadness, or frustration that comes with that. And that's OK. These feelings don't stay in their intense forms forever. They come and go like the tide, like labour contractions. They peak and they lessen in intensity. We can choose to ride the waves and recognise those emotions as valid.

Curbing the crash

Have you ever played that game with the fuel tank of your car? I have. The tank had been on red for a while. It has a handy countdown of miles. I began the journey with the notification saying there was under twenty miles remaining. I risked it. I kept thinking I'd visit the next petrol station but the kids were tired and hungry, so I kept chancing it for the next one.

Next it warned me that I had ten miles remaining. I glanced at the satnav to see that we were twelve miles from home. At one point, I was a couple of miles away from the nearest petrol station, and the car flashed up, '0 miles remaining'. My heart rate soared as I imagined having to call the car recovery people from the side of the road with an empty tank. I had sweaty palms as I drove the car onto the station forecourt. We barely made it. That could have been very frustrating.

Do you ever feel like you're playing that game with yourself? You brush off the call of your needs. You'll deal with them later. You'll deal with them another day. Maybe you'll deal with them never. Filling up with fuel and having slightly overtired and hungry kids would have been annoying. But standing on the side of the road in the grey drizzle would have been even more so.

I often say to clients, when we recognise that we are living with the red fuel light on, we have a choice. Refuel or grind to an inconvenient, messy halt at a time and place out of our control. Running on empty? Slow down, refuel, meet your needs or you'll get sick and burnt-out.

Think of your car. If you neglect the care of the tyres and the engine, it will run fine for a while until a warning light blinks for your attention. Overlook this and something will fall off or start to smoke. Neglect it further and it will no longer be able to take you from A to B.

I remember back when I was working crazy hours. I burnt the candle at both ends and then had to fit my life into weekends. I ended up getting flu that Christmas and it was hard to shake. I did too much for too long. I try to pace myself now. With the baby, I really need to do what I can to make sure I don't get wiped out again for that long.

Grace

We can recognise the need to look after something of value to us, such as a car. We can recognise this need in others, so why then does that recognition fade into insignificance when it comes to the caretaking of yourself? The car doesn't need to be squeaky clean, it needs the basic requirements met – fuel, water to cool the engine, the odd check over by a mechanic. Treating yourself like a machine is utterly unsustainable. You'll smoke and crash and something will fall off. Trust me, I've been there more times than I can count on both hands.

Numbing our needs

Have you got one of those washing machines that beep incessantly at you when it has finished its cycle? Wanting you to empty it so that the clean clothes don't become stagnant. You know what it requires. Yet what's the easiest thing to do when you've already got other stuff demanding your attention?

Switch the darn thing off.

You've stopped it shouting at you in its irritating, beeping way. But the need is still there. There is washing that needs to be taken out.

But at least it's quiet, right?

We do this with our own needs. Meeting them can feel inconvenient and another call on our time and energy. This is why we've simplified it by reaching for the warming glass of wine, some mindless scrolling or the TV remote. We can so easily turn to quick, easy fixes to satisfy our need for connection, space, comfort and stillness. We try to switch it off by numbing it. But the thing is, like the washing machine, the need is still there.

I'm meant to do these physio exercise things for my back. But by the time the kids are down, I honestly want to just sit on the sofa so

*I keep skipping them. I can feel it getting tighter and sorer. I really
do just need to do them for myself.*

Martha

Often the things that meet our needs require a bit more
energy. We don't always feel like we've got a lot of that to
go round. We can stop the washing machine beeping without sorting the issue. We're simply delaying it. And whilst
it's delayed, it becomes more urgent. The consequences of
ignoring it become higher as the hours and days go by. The
other option is that we can spend a few minutes dragging
the washing out and hanging it up.

If you're living life at 100 mph and ignoring your need to
take a breather, your tiredness isn't going to go away. It's going
to get worse as you turn your attention away from your body
to the other things that seem to be shouting louder.

Your needs are valid and valuable. Regardless of how
much validity and value you personally apply to them.

If you deem your children deserving of love and care.

Then you are deserving of it too.

That's a fact.

Self-care and self-sabotage

As you become more aware of what you need, recognise
that what might be self-care one day may be procrastination the next.

For example, putting the to-do list aside one day can be
an act of self-care. You know you need space and relief.

Time to rest when you'd usually be tearing round the house with the vacuum. Whereas, another day, putting the to-do list aside can be an act of self-sabotage. You avoid making the appointment you know you need to make or paying a bill. You avoid tidying whilst you can, so that you end up racing around even faster before your guests arrive on the Friday evening.

What might be self-care one day may be procrastination the next.

> *Sometimes I just sit down on the sofa and feel like I can't get up. Sometimes, that's good because I need to rest. Sometimes, it just makes things harder for myself later because there's stuff I genuinely need to do.*
>
> Helen

Self-care can be a large glass of wine in the sunshine or it can be forgoing the alcohol altogether. It can be taking a day of pyjama solitude, away from the world, or it might be ushering yourself out the door to socialise. Self-care might not even be a tangible 'thing' you do, but a new boundary you put in place in a tricky life-sapping relationship, or a text message asking for help. It's something that we need to be sensitive to so that we know how we need to respond to ourselves.

Start small, but start

Kick off that new cycle because you sure as hell can't pour from an empty cup. Don't wait until you 'feel' worth it to start making nurturing choices because it doesn't work that way round. Self-care cultivates self-worth. You need to introduce small, doable acts of self-care as a base requirement in line with brushing your teeth. It's about acknowledging your fundamental, innate worth and being able to give out to others safely.

Don't wait until you feel deserving of self-care to do it.

Go and indulge in a hot bath. And use the fancy stuff that you save for . . . I don't know. The queen? Well, I hate to say it but she's never coming. So . . .

Whether you make these changes for you, or you make them for them, it doesn't matter. Get that cog of low self-esteem turning in the opposite direction. Don't wait until you feel worth it. Start now, start small, but for the sake of your family and your mental health, start somewhere.

Some self-care prompts for you

To finish off, here are some prompts for self-care. One list is full of things you can fit into every day. They take almost no time at all, so no excuses. Some of them may seem basic and instinctive. But for many people, it's the basic things that get driven out and slip when we feel busy, burnt-out, low or overwhelmed. The second list contains some ideas for things that might take extra planning but will be worth it.

Daily self-care

- Drink water
- Go to the loo as soon as you need to
- Eat when hungry
- Brush your teeth
- Shower
- Get dressed
- Brush your hair
- Take your medication/vitamins on time
- Get outside
- Limit caffeine
- Read a couple of pages of a book
- Text a friend
- Floss
- Think of five things you are grateful for today
- Take ten deep breaths. Ensure the exhale is longer than the inhale
- Dab some diluted essential oil on your temple (try lavender)
- Drink warm soup from a mug (this was a game-changer when I wasn't fitting lunch in)
- Make your bed so you can climb in tonight
- Have a cup of herbal tea
- Do ten ten-second pelvic floor clenches
- Spend a couple of minutes doing some stretches
- Go to bed earlier

These might require some shuffling about of your day, or planning. But they will be worth it.

- Go for a brisk walk with the buggy or carrier
- Meet a friend for coffee
- Have a hot bath
- Use something you save for special occasions such as a nice bath oil, perfume or lipstick
- Take an extended shower and wash your hair
- Use a facemask
- Swap a social media scrolling session for a chapter of a book
- Download a guided meditation app and do a five–ten-minute meditation
- Exercise for ten–fifteen minutes
- Fill your fridge with some easy to grab, healthy, filling options
- Tick some things off your list that have been bothering you
- Do some stretching or yoga

Some of these acts of self-care seem boring, which they are. They are about meeting basic needs, which isn't fancy and fun, but can be really challenging for some. I'd like you to start implementing some non-negotiables to begin with. These might be eating when hungry, washing, drinking water or using the loo when you need to. Then begin to build on them, taking inspiration from the list and adding your own.

It can be helpful to journal your feelings around certain

self-care acts that you initially find challenging as it's encouraging to see how that changes.

Top Tip

Introduce one small act of self-care into your day, starting today.

JOURNAL POINTS

- What would you say about your level of self-care at the moment?
- What are your barriers to self-care?
- Name three things you need.
- What steps can you take to start to meet some of these needs?

Chapter 11

Tips and tools for easing anxiety

Mantra: *I am not made to do this alone.*

This is probably the part that you've been waiting for! This chapter is packed with tips and tools that will help with the symptoms of your anxiety. All the work you have done so far, to understand anxiety and explore how it impacts you, provides a foundation upon which to start using some techniques.

Because our experiences of anxiety vary, I'll share a host of techniques so that you'll find some that suit. Practise them when you are relaxed, so that they feel familiar for when anxiety next knocks at your door. Here is your toolkit. Whilst some of them may seem like small tools at first, they have the potential to shatter boulders.

Tip 1: Your breath is your superpower

It feels only right to begin with my absolute favourite technique. Breathing exercises.

I am fanatical about using the breath to address symptoms of anxiety. It has hands-down been the most important and simple technique I have ever added to my invisible, personal toolkit. I initially learnt about the impact that the breath can have on the nervous system at an antenatal class, before researching into how it can be used in other ways. I utilise it for so many things, from overtaking lorries and getting to sleep to dealing with toddler tantrums.

There are many different forms of breathing exercises you can do. I'm going to share with you my two favourites, but if these don't suit you for any reason, an internet video search will be able to talk you through some others.

1. Simple breathing exercise

This is a nice exercise to start with. If you find yourself feeling lightheaded or gasping for breath, stop the exercise and let your body return to its usual breath. Then try again later. Try practising with breathing through your nose only until you get used to it. We all have different lung capacities, so you might like to decrease each in- and out-breath by one count. The trick is to have a shorter inhale and an extended and full out-breath.

This exercise is brilliant for using throughout the day, as it doesn't require you to hold your breath and feels more instinctive. Isn't it amazing that you can be doing something to positively impact your nervous system and nobody would even know?

1.   Relax your jaw and drop your shoulders.

2.   Imagine filling your lungs from the bottom to the top to the count of four.
3.   Breathe out through your mouth to the count of eight.

Start with four repetitions and increase as you become more confident.

2. Breathing exercise with hold

The hold in this breathing exercise is intended to allow your body to make the most of the oxygen you've inhaled. The extra requirement to focus on the numbers can help distract your mind from the whirlwind of thoughts.

Be mindful that the breath-hold may take some getting used to. This is one to practise at home initially in case it makes you feel lightheaded. If so, shorten the counts on each step whilst you get used to it. Once you become more confident using this technique and your lungs adjust, you may find you can extend the timings of the exercise to suit you better.

1.   Relax your shoulders and your jaw.
2.   Breathe in through your nose gently and fully to the count of four. Imagine filling your lungs from the bottom to the top.
3.   Pause and hold your 'in' breath for the count of seven.
4.   Breathe out deeply through your mouth (purse your lips) to the count of eight.

Start with four repetitions and increase as you become more confident.

How does it work?

When we are anxious, we are likely to breathe more often and at a shallower rate. Do you notice yourself doing that? It's good to recognise because the more aware we can be, the sooner we can counteract it with a breathing exercise.

I hold my breath quite a bit when I feel stressed or anxious. I don't do it intentionally and I often realise because I have this tense feeling in my body or I hear myself take a sharp intake of breath. Both shallow breathing and breath holding are common **Shallow breathing and breath holding are common reactions to stress or anxiety.** reactions to stress or anxiety. We may also do either of them when we are nervous or anticipating something.

This interruption to our usual breathing rhythm activates the sympathetic nervous system, or stress, response. Breathing exercises essentially tell this physiological stress response to back down. This allows the parasympathetic nervous system to kick in. It says to your body, 'everything is OK. You aren't at threat.' And the body can step down from feeling like it is threatened. It's a physical response to what is often an internal trigger.

As you become more confident at using breathing exercises, you often end up becoming more sensitive to those earlier bubbles of anxiety. The ones that start to fizz up in response to a trigger or a fear. The earlier you respond to those first symptoms by using breath to calm the nervous system, the easier it will be to do so. It's much easier to fix a trickle of a tap leak than a full-blown burst pipe. And once you've calmed your body, you'll be more able to use your rational brain to address what is triggering your anxiety.

When I began using this technique, I would grab it in times of anxiety and stress. Sometimes I'd forget and sometimes I didn't feel I was doing it properly. I realised that I had to practise it so that I had the technique nailed for when I did need it. I practised it in the car, in the bath and before I went to sleep. As a result, it quickly became an instinctive reaction in those anxious moments. I could implement it earlier as the wave of anxiety came and it was much more effective. I use it without even thinking now, especially on the motorway when my anxiety and intrusive thoughts are commonly triggered. I also use it during stressful parenting moments as it gives me more chance of maintaining composure with grumpy children.

In my opinion, breathing exercises are beneficial for everyone experiencing anxiety. In fact, I utilise these breathing exercises most days, whether my feelings are anxiety-based or not. Breathing exercises work well to address difficult or intense emotions – stress, fear, anticipation, anger – that get the old sympathetic nervous system responding. They are also physically grounding and help us feel more present and able to engage in the moment.

I used a breathing exercise this morning during a few particularly testing moments. In all honesty, the whole morning was one long testing 'moment'. When I feel stress rise in my body like the swell of a tide, I use these techniques to breathe it back down. I'm not doing it to ignore feelings or devalue them, I'm telling my body that it's safe.

Breathing exercises – I totally underestimated them until my friend told me they'd helped her stop a few panic attacks. I started to practise them and now use them all the time. Even when I'm not feeling anxious, I use them to relax myself. It's like a life hack. We all need to do it.

Anna

Breathing for panic attacks

If you suffer panic attacks, you'll be familiar with some of the symptoms that the sympathetic nervous system response evokes. People speak of increased heart rate, sweating, a sense of difficulty breathing and shaking. I remember my first panic attack, about twelve years ago. I thought I was having a heart attack. I felt totally helpless to what was happening in my body. Many an ambulance has been sent to help a person who believed they were having a heart attack but were actually having a panic attack. Such is the strength of the experience and the fear it can evoke.

The important thing to know is that, whilst they can feel overwhelming, panic attacks aren't dangerous. It's a physical response to stress, danger or even excitement. If you've experienced a panic attack, you may have felt spaced out and disconnected from the world. It may have sounded like people's voices were far away. Or you may have felt like your surroundings were quickly closing in. The body and brain are so intricately connected, leading to many strange sensations and emotions.

Whilst they can feel overwhelming, panic attacks aren't dangerous.

If you experience panic attacks, breathing exercises are a brilliant tool. The trick is to become so familiar with your chosen breathing exercise that you implement it automatically.

I've got so good now at starting the breathing exercises when I feel the panic coming on. I used to try when it had already hit and that's a bit harder really. It works very well. I used to think it was impossible to control.

Sheetal

When our anxiety is triggered, our brain tells our body that we're at threat. Our sympathetic nervous system, fight or flight, stress response kicks in. Then we feel the physical effects of this stress response, which can trigger further fear. This fear fuels the stress response. The physical symptoms fuel the fear. And then we find ourselves caught inside the anxiety wave, tumbling over and over, feeling like we are going to suffocate.

If you experience panic attacks, you've survived them all to this day. My hope is that the chapters you've read will have given you some good insight into the workings of your anxiety, so that you may be better equipped to recognise what sparks your panic attacks.

Breathing for sleep

You've got a baby, so it's likely that your sleep quality isn't at its finest anyway. You may be awake feeding, administering teething remedies or due to any other of the many reasons they have us up in the dark hours. However, you don't need your anxiety to be yet another reason to be exhausted when morning breaks.

Anxiety can impact our sleep. I've spent many an hour playing out scenarios in my mind, worrying and over-analysing. This activates our physical stress response, as we know, and this is a state of arousal. Not the sexy kind, it's the alert, gotta-keep-my-wits-about-me kind. Think back to the caveman, if he knows he's at threat, and there's a bear roaming the woods, he's not going to sleep deeply. His body is primed to protect his family and food sources.

This state of arousal is not conducive to sleep. Oh no! Cortisol, the stress hormone, will cause you to be wakeful and alert when you would rather be resting. Signs that this is happening may be that you struggle to fall asleep, you wake fully at night or you wake early in the morning.

Breathing exercises are brilliant for sleep as they activate the parasympathetic nervous system, which is also termed 'the rest and digest' response. In time, this can help lower the caffeine-like cortisol fizzing around your body. It also helps to use the breathing exercises throughout the day, so that when you get to bed, you are hopefully already experiencing a lower physiological stress level.

I use breathing exercises before I go to sleep. I do a 'body scan' where I relax a bit of my body at a time and then I do my deep breathing exercise. I fall asleep really quickly like this. When my little girl wakes me up, I do it again, especially if I'm totally wide awake.

Flora

Other things that use a grounding breath

I found swimming really helped quieten my mind and calm my body. I didn't quite understand why at first because it's an active thing to do. But then I realised that the rhythmic breathing you do when you swim front crawl is like the exercises we've discussed. You take a deep inhale, and then your exhale is full and long as you complete some strokes.

Yoga, meditation and all swimming strokes utilise this type of breath in action. As a result, they are quickly becoming my favourite ways to ground myself when life feels a bit like a whirlwind. Should you want to use the breath you've been practising in a slightly different context, there are so many guided practices online. Please check that any exercise is suitable for you in this postnatal period.

I did some pregnancy yoga. I only went to meet other mums really. But it was so helpful and relaxing. I used the breathing during my c-section. I try to do five minutes a day now before I go to bed as there's something about it that makes me feel better in myself.

Sasha

Tip 2 – Vital vulnerability

Vulnerability is a non-negotiable tool if you ask me. It should be one of your toolbox staples. I can't stress the absolute importance of vulnerability. It takes practice, it needs to be strengthened and nurtured. It changed my life. Let me explain.

You are simply not created to do this thing called motherhood alone. Not mentally, not physically. Trust me, I tried for years to keep my challenges with my

Vulnerability is a non-negotiable tool.

mental health to myself, and it was nothing but exhausting and unsustainable. I'm sure you've tried for a long time to 'sort this anxiety/worry out' using your own strength and resources.

Vulnerability often gets a bad rap because people associate it with weakness and messiness. It used to make me think of a tiny bird that had fallen out of its nest and broken its wing. These days, when I think of vulnerability, I think of courage and strength. To be vulnerable is to be authentic to who we are, where we've come from, and where we are in our journey.

I found it so hard to talk about the stuff I was anxious about. To be honest, I never did. But one day I opened up to a friend randomly. I'm not even sure why. I was so worried she'd think I was crazy but she was so understanding and shared stuff she'd been feeling too. It made such a difference to how I felt, just knowing that someone knew and understood.

Jas

The vulnerability drawbridge

One of the biggest boundaries to allowing others insight into your inner world is when you've been let down previously. Perhaps you've taken the risk to open up to someone you hoped would understand or support you but you didn't get the response you'd yearned for.

Being let down or misunderstood undeniably dents our confidence and desire to seek support again. I personally find it hard when I feel misunderstood after I've tried to voice something that matters to me, be it an opinion or a feeling. That's because I take it personally, as if that person is making a statement about the invalidity of how I feel. I have to remind myself that not everyone will understand how I feel.

People may say and do unhelpful things in response to your openness. This is more likely to be due to a lack of understanding or differing life experience, than a reflection on you.

Sometimes we avoid being vulnerable with others because of previous hurt or because our vulnerability has been abused in some way. It's then easy to make self-protective, blanket assumptions that everyone else will respond badly too.

My ex-partner would manipulate the stuff I'd told him in confidence and use it against me in arguments. It really made me want to shut down and not be open with people.

Anonymous

We find ourselves building tall emotional walls and barriers to keep people out. The issue is, that whilst we may feel emotionally protected, we also end up keeping out those who could be the ones to make a difference. It's a safe place behind the wall but it sure can feel lonely there.

Vulnerability is a risk. When I first knew I had to open up about the reality of how I felt whilst in the depths of my postnatal anxiety and depression, I was scared. I was worried that people would deem me an unfit mother, brand me 'mad' or take my baby away. I feared that friends would avoid me. I didn't want to be a burden. I was worried my family would worry (I see the irony in that sentence now).

And you know, not everyone understood. I remember one friend proclaiming, 'Anna, you're so lucky. Focus on the fact you have a baby and many people can't. Be happy.' Whilst well intended I'm sure, her response worked to compound my sense of guilt and shame. Whilst she is a wonderful friend, I simply determined that she probably wasn't the best person to speak to about that part of my life. The temptation was to shut down and not speak to anyone else out of fear of them having the same response. But I did speak to someone else. And then I spoke to someone else. And then I spoke to someone else. And now I'm speaking to you. And I'm glad I risked it.

Sometimes, someone will respond in a way that makes you feel totally and utterly heard and your feelings valid. Once we feel like we can be open with someone about how we're feeling, it enables us to access the support and compassion we need. In addition, it builds our confidence in sharing our story.

There's nothing like feeling understood.

Priya

There is no way I'd have believed you if you'd told me I'd one day be typing up some of my deepest and darkest thoughts for you to read. I would have been filled with shame and fear at what you'd think. This is the impact of sharing our stories. We realise that just because not everyone understands our experience, it doesn't mean it's invalid.

I've shared my story so many times, although perhaps not to the depth I have here. But I've also been party to the inner lives of so many women who have consulted me as a therapist. I *know* we are not alone. I *know* that our darkest thoughts do not deserve to be shrouded in the shame we keep them in. Silence keeps us stuck. Vulnerability with the right people enables us to access freedom and hope.

Who should I speak to?

Your support network doesn't have to be big. It would be exhausting to update a host of friends on how you are. In an ideal world, one of these would be your partner because in theory they know you best. Another might be a close friend.

Speak to someone who knows you well, who has been supportive, kind and warm in the past. Another person may be a mental health professional, such as a GP or therapist. Or someone you've met in an online support group. I underestimated the strength I could gain from online support until I was invited to join a Facebook group of women expecting their babies at the same time as me. Those women were invaluable to my mental health journey. Somehow it felt easier to pour my words out into a message rather than verbalise them.

I've got lots of 'friends' but only, maybe three of them really, really know me well. But that's how I like it. That's healthy for me.

Alison

Little by little

You don't need to tell everyone everything. You might not believe it but it's actually a huge privilege to be let into your internal world. Think about how you feel when a friend opens up about something you know means a lot to them. It tends to feel like an honour and a responsibility to be let in. It's often a challenge to believe that others may feel this way about you.

You don't need to tell everyone everything.

Take small steps towards opening up with those you feel have the potential to be trustworthy. See what happens each time you take a tiny step of vulnerability with that person. If they are the right person, and respond supportively, it will increase your confidence in sharing further.

When a friend opens up to me, I feel so lucky and touched that they felt able to tell me things that not everyone else knows.

Bec

Knowing what you need

It's all very well encouraging you to be open with people but what happens when you don't know what it is that you need from them. Is it advice? Perhaps it's comfort, a hug, a listening ear, to be made to laugh or some practical support?

What do you need?

Right now? What do you need?

From a friend, from this book, from your partner?

Do you know? Is that an easy question for you to answer?

I remember being asked a few years ago by a kindly lecturer. She was so sincere. She really wanted me to ask myself what I needed. It made me cry. I cried because I didn't know.

It wasn't that I didn't need anything, I did. I simply hadn't considered my needs because I'd been so focused on meeting and pre-empting the needs of others. That's where I got my sense of worth from because my self-esteem was so low at that point. I cried because I suddenly realised that I had no clarity on what the tangled ball of unmet, unspoken, unheard need in my stomach was.

Perhaps you are also so focused on meeting the needs of those around you, and tending to their feelings, that you don't even know the language of your own. Obviously, that is what motherhood is. It's responsibility for monitoring the wellbeing of a tiny person. But it certainly doesn't call us to ignore our own. Just because suddenly you are responsible for someone of immense value, it doesn't then mean that you are worthless. Your needs are as important. Sure, maybe they can't always be met (a week's sleep please) and sometimes they have to wait (screaming baby fed, then I sort my rumbling tummy) but, ultimately, they deserve to be acknowledged too.

I started to eat proper lunch because I realised I was feeding the baby good food and just snacking on stuff for myself. I wanted her to see me eat good meals too so that when she's older, she'll know it's important.

Federica

Fear, feeling, need

Anxiety can be an umbrella feeling for other emotions that we aren't quite aware of or in touch with.

Imagine anxiety as a prism. One beam of light goes into one side and then refracts, casting a rainbow of colour over the wall. Anxiety is like the plain white light. It feels like a feeling, whereas it is trying to tell us a story. It is trying to express unmet, unheard and unspoken fears, feelings and needs. Therefore, if we're going to try to start meeting them through self-care and vulnerability, it's good to start asking ourselves what those might actually be.

How am I feeling?

This isn't always an easy one to answer when you first begin. Try on some feelings like clothes. Name them to yourself and see if they fit. Am I hungry, lonely, frustrated, tired, cold, thirsty, sad, hurt, angry?

What do I need?

Do you need anything in response to the feeling you've named? Perhaps you need reassurance, food, rest, a good chat or to say 'no' to something. It would be brilliant if you could act on it in some way, even if it's small, even if it's simply an acknowledgment.

And when you feel anxious, ask yourself:

What am I fearing?

Can you identify what has triggered you? Which tool can you use in order to help re-anchor and re-ground yourself?

Maybe you need to step out and take a breather for a moment or call a friend to hear a reassuring voice.

The more we suppress these things deep down inside, the more emotional and physiological stress we will be under. And, the more likely these feelings are to get displaced onto something else, for example feelings of grief might turn into anxiety about health or obsessive-compulsive behaviour in order to avoid death. You know when you're upset or angered by something but end up crying or losing your rag about something else unrelated to the actual issue? That's displacement.

I want you to start checking in with yourself at least twice a day. Set it as a reminder on your phone. Write it in eyeliner on your mirror.

What am I feeling? Do I need anything? As you become more able to answer these questions, you'll get to know yourself better. Maybe you'll start to see patterns or identify triggers. Insight is such an incredible tool as it allows us to pre-empt, prepare and equip ourselves for next time. Much of how anxiety impacts us is based around the feeling of helplessness, like it's happening to us. Ultimately, we have more control than we realise. Understanding what lies beneath our anxious feelings is so helpful.

I barely ever think about what I am worried about or feeling, it just comes out when I'm in bed and I stop.

                                                                Sally

Tip 3 – Switching up your thought habits

We're going to look at common ways of thinking that take up precious headspace. These are the fast-track rides to finding yourself amidst an anxiety whirlwind. You'll be equipped with tools to help you for when you find yourself focusing on what could go wrong, overthinking and avoidance.

Have an attitude of gratitude

Now, before I talk about gratitude, I want to say that we can feel many things in tandem. Happiness and grief. Confusion and clarity. Gratitude isn't a call to be constantly happy and always looking at the bright side of life (are you now singing that too?). It can be an amazing tool for shifting focus from anxious thoughts about what could go wrong to what has gone right and what is good.

Gratitude shifts the focus from what could go wrong to what has gone right.

Gratitude introduces balance when we have tipped into negativity. It can remind us of the light when we have been gazing at the dark greys. I've got two simple exercises that I use regularly to really challenge my mindset when I've got into a slump, a rut or a spiral. For me, they can be transformational. They can completely U-turn my thoughts and lift my feelings.

1. Reframe the mundane

When you find yourself bogged down with the day-to-day grind, the to-do list, the worries and frustrations, change 'I've got to' to 'I get to'.

'I've got to do three loads of washing', turns into . . .

'I get to do three loads of washing.'

What went from a chore, turns into a privilege. I have a washing machine. I'm incredibly lucky! I have a family. My children have clothes to wear. I'm not entitled to any of that. I'm so fortunate. So often when I've used this technique, I've gone from shoving and stuffing clothes into machines and baskets, to feeling tearful because I'm looking at the garments my children wear; my children, their clothes, our privilege.

I use this a lot. I get to do the nursery run. I get to drive them in our car, through the winding countryside, from our home to a nursery and school where they're taught. I get to see their small legs walking. I get to hold their hands. I get to pop to the supermarket on the way home to buy food for our dinner.

This is not about batting away what are valid and natural feelings that come with living in the chaos of family life and motherhood. It sure can feel tiring, relentless and tear-filled at times. That's OK! But it feels so good to view it with gratitude. I find it really anchors and grounds me and I hope it may do the same for you too.

2. Gratitude list

Every day, list things you're grateful for. It doesn't matter whether you do it in your mind before you go to sleep, on the back of a napkin or in a daily journal. Note five things you are grateful for. They can range from the momentous to the seemingly insignificant.

A brilliant challenge is to write a list of 100 things you are grateful for! It's easier than it sounds once you get on a roll. You start with big things like family, your baby. And then as you continue, you end up really feeling grateful for the small things that really aren't that small at all. The fact you're sitting on a chair, the fact you can write, see, walk to find a pen in a home that keeps you warm.

When we are caught in a whirlwind of anxiety or negativity, it can be hard to see the wood for the trees. Gratitude helps draw our attention and focus to the diamonds that can be found amidst the murky watery sand.

Honestly, practising gratitude has the ability to totally transform my day and mood. I wish I had started doing it earlier. It's has changed me into a glass half-full person.

Ella

Put the brakes on overthinking

Overthinking is often sparked by a tiny fear-based thought or feeling that we don't even realise we've had. When we take hold of that thought and begin to overthink, it's like pouring fuel slowly onto a flickering ember. In hardly any time at all, the spark has turned into a roaring, consuming fire. We are then left to wonder how on earth we went from feeling calm into a full-blown head spin.

> *I get one thought and then it grows and grows until I feel like it's certainly going to happen. It's scary how quickly thoughts can change my whole mindset.*
>
> Makayla

It can feel like you don't have control over this thought spiral. It's like the rollercoaster carriage that has been pushed off the highest point and gathers unstoppable speed as it hurtles down the track. You have more control than your mind will lead you to believe. You are not at the mercy of your thoughts. Overthinking is a habit, a way of dealing with anxious thoughts that has become a way of life. Fortunately, we can change our habits. It will take time to strengthen the mental muscles that stop the spiralling but it can be done. Don't forget that you'll be more susceptible to falling into spirals when your energy or resources are depleted in any way.

Here are three techniques you might like to try.

1. Write the thoughts down on paper. Sometimes seeing things in black and white, and outside your own mind, can bring clarity and perspective. It can allow you to rationalise things more easily.
2. When you notice yourself spiralling into overthinking, ask yourself what the facts are. This can be really grounding and can bring your scattered, creative mind back into focus.

For example, your baby has been taken out by her grandparents for a couple of hours. Instead of getting some jobs done and then relaxing as instructed, you have found yourself in a tailspin of worry and you can't focus. What if something happens? What if they feed her an unsliced grape and she chokes? What if they forget to strap the car seat in properly and they crash? (I've thought *all* these things.)

Right. Let's look at the facts. Her grandparents have so far always been vigilant. She will get far more focused attention than if she were at home whilst you were doing jobs. They love her too and want her to be safe and happy. You've shown them how to strap the car seat in. You can drop them a quick text reminder to halve the grapes in the picnic as you forgot to say. They will be back soon. Nothing bad happened last time.

Our brains like to fill in the gaps. And if we're feeling anxious, what our brain fills the gaps in with will be reflective of our anxiety. Be grounded by the facts. Use the breathing exercises you've learnt to calm your body's fear response.

3. As soon as you notice your mind overthinking like a runaway train, say 'STOP' out loud or in your mind. Then find a way to fill up your mind with something else. Perhaps you count backwards from 100 in threes or recite a times table. Or maybe sing your favourite song. I often use maths as a distraction technique because I'm not that good at it, so it requires focus and effort. When we are focusing with effort on something, our thoughts can't spiral. We don't have the ability to feed both maths

calculations and the whirlwind of creative, fear-based scenarios.

The more often you utilise these techniques, the more habitual they will become.

Become your own coach

We've chatted about internal dialogue a fair bit now (see Chapter 9 for more on this) and hopefully you've become increasingly confident at tweaking and challenging it. Now I want you to think about how you can use that internal dialogue to coach you through anxious moments.

Imagine a brilliant, supportive person who is also firm, but in a loving way. They are kind, compassionate and experienced. You might be thinking of a particular person right now, someone you actually know. Use their voice and hold them in mind when you are coaching yourself. Imagine what they would say and how they would guide you if they knew what was going on in your mind. It is also effective to conjure up an imaginary person or perhaps you want to think about what I would say to you. It doesn't matter. What's important is that you can imagine someone in your mind who is a separate entity to the thoughts you have.

Use this voice to coach you through anxious moments. Perhaps you are taking your baby for a round of jabs and your thoughts are spiralling about side effects and seeing your baby uncomfortable. Your internal coach might say something like, 'It's OK. I'm here. I know it's hard but you're doing what you feel is best for him. Breathe through it and he will also feel you relax. Babies have this done all the time. In a few minutes, he won't remember the feeling of the needle. If there are any side effects you are worried about, you can call the doctor. Everyone wants you both to feel safe. You've got this.'

I literally pep talk myself when I'm having a wobble. I imagine what my best mate would say to me if she was there. It's so good!
                                                                Mary

Like with all these new habits you're forming, be kind to yourself. It may well feel like a faltering whisper at first. As you start to use it more it will grow in authority, volume and immediacy.

Ensure that your inner coach is warm, kind and firm. Not strict and irritable. As frustrated as you may feel about your anxiety, a strict or bullying response isn't going to beat anxiety into submission; it is only going to feed it.

Addressing avoidance

One way we might have dealt with our challenging thought patterns is to avoid our triggers. It's human nature to want to avoid what makes us feel anxious, stressed or unhappy. If our mind and body has learnt that something is anxiety provoking, it is more likely to trigger that fight or flight sympathetic nervous system response.

The challenge comes when we are being triggered by day-to-day events such as weaning our babies or socialising. When we are feeling tempted to avoid something that in and of itself isn't dangerous, we can limit our lives. We can end up avoiding what may be life enriching when we avoid something altogether, or keep removing ourselves from the situation as soon as we sense the anxiety rolling in.

When we remove ourselves from a situation as soon as we feel anxious, our anxiety is reinforced for the next time we are faced with the triggering situation. I'm talking about situations that we feel threatened by for some reason but that aren't threatening. I use this technique often when my anxiety is triggered and my temptation is to leave a busy playgroup full of people I don't know or turn down an invitation because I don't fancy the motorway.

If we find a way to ride the wave of anxiety whilst staying in the triggering situation, then we will begin to reinforce a new message. This new message will be that we can do it; we can endure it and come out alive and proud. Your anxiety may have you believe that the physical and mental symptoms will increase and increase into oblivion. But physiologically that isn't possible.

It can feel like your anxious thoughts and feelings will rise indefinitely. But it's more like a wave or a labour contraction that has a peak, and then falls. We dismantle the trigger-anxiety association by arming ourselves with the right tools to enable us to ride that wave without jumping off the surfboard and climbing into the lifeboat. As you glide onto the beach off the rocky wave, you feel immensely proud of yourself. You *can* surf that wave after all.

If you looked at your anxiety on a graph whilst staying in your triggering situation, even without any intervention or breathing exercises, the line will increase to an apex. That may be a full-blown panic attack. And then it will start to decrease as your worst fears aren't realised, and your mind realises it's not in full threat, as it had believed.

I passionately detest spiders. My anxiety spikes when I see one and everything in me wants to escape. I've had the postman come in to remove one before. My husband usually deals with them when he's around but the other day, there was a huge one in the kitchen. He was at work. I needed to get the kids breakfast.

Whilst the temptation was to shut the door, burn the house down and take the kids out to nursery and school unfed ... I had to deal with it. With shaking hands, I got the vacuum cleaner, faked my confidence (I don't want the kids to be scared of them too ... I want them to be able to remove them for me in years to come. Ha ha!). I'm sorry if you're a pacifist but I sucked the spider up and calmly put (ahem, threw) the appliance in the garage should it be able to crawl back out.

Once I had breathed down the pace of my galloping heart and wiped my sweaty palms on my pyjamas, I felt immensely proud of myself. I'd had no choice but to ride the wave of anxiety but, as it abated, my confidence grew. I had another spider encounter shortly afterwards, when one casually sauntered across the rug whilst I was watching TV. My husband was out. I felt the familiar spike of anxiety but I knew I could handle it because I had handled it before. Fact. I gave it a very wide berth as I grabbed my faithful vacuum. Each time I do this, my confidence increases, my anxiety doesn't spike quite so high and my heart rate settles quicker. It works.

Set yourself bite-sized challenges. When you feel your

anxiety rise, use the techniques, look at the clock and try to stick it out for a few more minutes. You know what your victories are. Celebrate them, no matter how small, and use them to encourage yourself next time you are faced with your trigger. There is so much more for you than living a life consumed with fear. You may find it helpful to find a friend, family member or therapist to support you and help you remain anchored as the peak of anxiety passes.

I had therapy for my fear of heights because I was worried about passing it on to my son. I was encouraged to challenge myself by exposing myself to various heights. What really helped was to stay there until I felt calm. Now I still feel anxious but I just breathe and I'm so proud of myself.

Megan

Tip 4 – Pick 'n' mix grounding exercises

You might want to turn over the corner of this page as it's a good one to flip back to when you need it. It's like a sweetie shop of grounding exercises – a pick 'n' mix. Try one, see if you like it, see if it works for you. If not, try another. Once you get into grabbing these, you may even find yourself making up new ones that suit you even better.

Grounding exercises are like magnets for the mind. They draw back all the scattered thoughts whizzing around, causing your head to spin and your heart to race. They bring you back into the present moment where the solid ground is. They enable you to access your rational brain more easily, to determine the hard facts over the creative possibilities.

It's good to remind yourself that you can't be both fully present and engaged in the current moment, whilst also contemplating 100 other anxiety-provoking scenarios. Your brain doesn't have the capacity to do both.

Here is your pick 'n' mix. Everyone has different tastes according to how we think and process things, but there will be something to suit you.

Mind fillers

- Five-four-three-two-one. From where you are standing or sitting, name five things you can see, four things you can touch, three things you can hear, two things you can smell and one thing you can taste.
- Look around and find things beginning with each letter of the alphabet.
- Attempt mathematical sums or count back from 100 in threes.
- Try to recite the alphabet backwards.
- Read a few pages of a book, put on a song you love or play a quick game of something on your phone that requires concentration or logic.

Physical grounding

- Breathe in for four, out for eight.
- Put your feet flat on the floor and imagine tree roots

reaching down into the earth. Rub your palms together
and feel them warming.

- Splash cool water on your wrists, neck or face. Notice
  how it feels and describe the sensations to yourself.
- Make a hot drink. Concentrate on all the noises,
  sensations, smells and actions.

*When I start overthinking, I distract myself by adding together the
birth dates of my family. It sounds silly but it does stop me from
overthinking really well.*

Shaz

Going to your safe place

Just as your child may have a comforter that they turn to
when they are feeling worried or insecure, we can create
an adult version. Do you have anything in your life that
evokes a feeling of comfort or safety? It might be a thing,
such as a soft stone you found on a beach during a happy
holiday. Perhaps you have a piece of jewellery you associate with someone kind and comforting. It can be helpful
to keep that thing close for you to touch or hold when
you need it.

Alternatively, you can use a memory of a place you felt
calm and secure. Imagine it now and recall the colours,
noises and smells. When you feel your mind wandering and
anxious, draw it back to that safe and comfortable place.

*I used to play in the woods at the back of the house by a tiny
stream. Some of my happiest memories were made there. When*

I'm stressed, I imagine being there when the sun was shining and I felt happy.

Aimee

Tip 5 – Helpful lifestyle tweaks

Often my clients are surprised when I ask them a few questions about their lifestyle. They have come to me to talk about their mind, so some of my questions may, at first, seem somewhat irrelevant.

It is so important to explore your lifestyle when addressing your mental health. The most powerful shifts come when we explore things holistically, from different angles. It's easy to focus on the 'thinking', but the lifestyle choices we make can feed into, or help reduce, symptoms of anxiety.

Diet

Diet has a strong impact on our mental health and emotions. In this way, our emotions can also drive the decisions we make about food. Think about how the food choices you make differ when you feel happy, low, hormonal, tired, healthy, self-accepting or frustrated. It's good to be aware of this so that you can give yourself the opportunity to make decisions that may not exacerbate your feelings.

When I'm tired or feeling low, I seek sugar highs. I want quick fixes that lift me physically. I want the burst of energy and that satisfying hit of the pleasure chemical dopamine that comes with sugary food. Things feel better for a bit.

After the sugar high comes the sugar crash and it's not so pretty. It's a depressive crash that can make you feel shaky, tired, low and irritable. Then I feel as low as before, if not more so, because I now feel physically depleted as well as mentally. The temptation then, for me, is to scour the cupboards for my next temporary fix.

If you recognise this cycle seek balanced meals containing proteins, fats and complex carbohydrates. It might be the last thing on your mind as you reach into the cupboard but ask yourself if you want to make yourself feel better or ultimately worse. Your taste buds don't care about your mental state. My kids would happily live on sweet treats but I care more about their bodies than they do. I have to make grown-up decisions for them. Sometimes we need that inner coach to step in.

I won't make particular dietary recommendations as I'm not qualified, but please speak to a medical or dietary practitioner, or do some research into dietary changes that might stabilise your blood sugar.

I find coffee so warming, reassuring and energising. I feel my heart rate increase. I feel more alert and focused. My tiredness gets temporarily blurred over. However, your caffeine intake is also something to monitor. I'm such a buzz-kill but if you're prone to anxiety, it's important to know that caffeine triggers the release of adrenaline and stimulates the nervous system. It's the same hormone behind the fight or flight response that you experience with anxiety.

Keep an eye on how you feel when you've had caffeine. See if you recognise an increase in anxious thoughts or feelings afterwards, or on the days you have more. The physical effects of drinking caffeine can trigger anxious thoughts, just as anxious thoughts can trigger the physical feelings. If you notice a link at all, then you may need to decrease or halt your caffeine intake.

If you do decide to cut down, try to wean off slowly rather than going cold turkey

Keep an eye on how you feel when you've had caffeine.

to lessen sudden withdrawal headaches and aches. (I've learnt the hard way. I thought I was coming down with flu.) If it's the warmth or the ceremony of making a hot drink that you enjoy, try replacing a cup or two with herbal tea.

> *I only drink one cup of tea a day now. I cut down when I was pregnant and it made me feel way less anxious in my chest. That fluttery feeling calmed down.*
>
> Frankie

Engage in a higher power

Many people find that engaging in a 'higher power' can be positive for their mental health. A belief or faith in something bigger than ourselves, and outside ourselves, can be a source of strength.

Over the years I've worked with addiction, many of my clients have engaged in twelve-step programmes such as Alcoholics Anonymous or Narcotics Anonymous. It was common for them to feed back that having a higher power had been a very important factor in their recovery. Who their higher power is doesn't matter so much as the sense of connection, strength, peace and purpose they draw from it. Engaging in faith-based communities, meditating, praying or carrying out positive rituals can provide a holistic approach to anxiety and mental health challenges.

If spirituality or religion are important to you, you might like to explore ways to integrate it within your approach to addressing your anxiety. If it has been a positive influence in your life in the past, then maybe you'd consider re-engaging.

I pray every day, and more when things are hard. I like knowing I can pray whenever I like. I feel like God is listening to me and giving me strength.

Anonymous

Exercise

Don't switch off to me quite yet! I know you're tired and the juggle can be a struggle. But I'll be sensible and realistic with what I recommend, I promise.

Exercise is one of my favourite tools for addressing my mental health. It undoubtedly benefits us physically but the mental benefits are incredible. Exercise encourages growth of neurons in the brain, reduces blood pressure and releases endorphins (feel-good chemicals). It can also act as good distraction for whirlwind thoughts. What's more, it releases tension, relaxes muscles, improves sleep so that what sleep you do manage to get is likely to be better quality. All of these things increase your sense of general wellbeing and positively influence mental health.

My mental health really benefits when I include exercise

into my day. I'm talking about a quick five-minute yoga video whilst the baby sleeps or a walk around the block. I may not be able to accommodate the long gym sessions of yester-year but that doesn't mean that five, ten or twenty minutes of exercise are pointless. Anything that gets your heart rate raised slightly is perfect.

I am one of those mums who spend much of the day in activewear, taking the first opportunity to fit in a bit of exercise. I often get up before the kids and do it then, and have been known not to shower and get out of my gear until bedtime. When I feel low, exercise is one of the first things I put back into my routine. I never regret it, as it doesn't fail to give me the boost I need. Even a few minutes helps my mindset.

Start small – maybe with a brisk walk or a ten-minute postnatal exercise video from the comfort of your lounge. When we feel shattered by life, motherhood and the day-to-day juggle, we often lack motivation, therefore, taking that first small step is necessary to break that cycle. Try it a few times a week and see if it positively impacts your mental health.

I swear, my exercise is like therapy. I have always done it three times a week. I feel mentally different when I don't do it because it really lifts my mood. I do it while George sleeps.

Sophie

Get outside

It's good to set the goal of going outside at least once per day. There is more and more research being published suggesting that spending time in nature reduces feelings of anxiety, stress and depression. The other day, after being indoors writing and juggling kids, as soon as my husband came home I dashed out for a quick ten-minute stride around the block. My mind went from fuzzy to refreshed. In fact, I should probably take a break and dash out now.

Maybe it's time to get your trainers on, stick on some uplifting music or a podcast, and get out there. I often drag the tired boys off the sofa late afternoon to head out for a quick walk or scoot. Florence has her last nap in the carrier and we all come back rosy cheeked. It's one of those things that's so easy not to do, it's a faff to usher the kids into jackets and helmets when they'd rather watch TV. But it makes such a difference when we do.

Go with the flow

Have you recently been so immersed and in the flow of something that you've lost track of time? We can feel this way when doing something creative. Maybe you get that feeling when reading, playing games or chatting with a good friend. We forget the wider world around us and time melts away as if it's not a thing at all. When we're in the flow, all that seems to exist is the present moment.

It's harder to find time to do these activities when we've got so many calls on our attention. But these 'flow' activities are thought to bring stress relief and increase a sense of wellbeing. Is there something you used to love doing that you could find a way to reintroduce into your life? Perhaps you can grab your knitting needles back out or a colouring book. Swap some online scrolling or TV time with a flow activity and see how you feel afterwards.

Someone bought me a colouring book for my birthday. I find it really relaxing even though my husband laughs at me. I could do it for hours!

Laura

Thoughts on medication

I regularly get asked my opinion on medication. Whether you should take it, stop it, increase it or reduce it. That is for you to discuss with your doctor. They know your full medical history and any contraindications that may impact your decisions.

However, I do have a couple of tips that will be helpful for you if you are taking or considering anti-anxiety medications:

1. Think about how you are feeling and set a timeline of a week or two depending on the intensity of your anxiety (less time for higher intensity). In that time commit to prioritising and consistently employing some of your favourite grounding exercises and tips. I recommend that you include addressing your internal dialogue, breathing exercises and being more open about your emotions with your select few.

   At the end of that time period, re-evaluate how you're feeling. If you've not seen any relief or positive shift, prioritise scheduling a chat with your doctor.

Regardless of whether you choose to take medication or not, continue using the tools and techniques as they will support you too.

2. If you take anti-anxiety medication, it is most effective when used alongside the techniques and tips we've discussed. These tools will be aiding you in addressing the mental and physical elements of anxiety. Plus, as you use the techniques that help you, they will become even more engrained to support you when or if you choose to reduce or halt your medication.

Imagine that you have a badly sprained ankle and need crutches to get around. You use the crutches to allow you to resume daily life as much as you can. They remove the weight from your foot to give it rest. However, life on crutches isn't the end goal. Your physiotherapist gives you certain repetitive exercises to build muscle tone and strength. This means that when the crutches are removed, you have built up the strength to walk. The crutches are the medication and the techniques are like the physiotherapy exercises. They intend to build your confidence and increase your level of insight.

Being honest with people and taking time to rest have made such a difference to how I feel. So I needed to do them more when I lowered my medication dosage.

Anonymous

Top Tip

Next time you start overthinking, try to recite the alphabet backwards.

JOURNAL POINTS

- What techniques have helped you in the past?
- After reading this chapter, which techniques or lifestyle tweaks will you try?
- When and how will you practise them? What can you do to remind yourself?
- Try one of the breathing exercises for ten rounds.
- Can you notice any changes in your mind or body afterwards?

Chapter 12

Slow and steady

Mantra: *This is going to be worth it.*

And we reach the final chapter! I'm going to use these pages to cheerlead you. To encourage you to persevere regardless of how quickly you see the benefits. You are forming habits that will benefit you for life. The good stuff takes time. We are used to speed. We receive shopping on our doorstep mere hours after clicking 'buy', and food handed to us minutes after ordering. But you can't grow a baby in a day, nurture a marriage or deepen a friendship so quickly. No, the good, life-changing stuff takes time.

So this chapter is full of encouragement, advice on setbacks and some heartfelt words from me to you.

Your work on anxiety is never in vain

Addressing anxiety is like tapping away at a huge ten-foot block of ice. You're standing beside it, tapping away with a tiny silver toffee hammer. You long to see the ice shatter to the ground so you can do a victory dance upon the melting shards.

Every time you speak back to that familiar, cruel voice, you're tapping with that hammer. No matter how successful it was, I encourage you pick it up again next time too. Each time, you're tapping that block of ice. Yes, maybe sometimes introduce a new or additional tool, especially as they slowly become second nature and less effort, but make sure you always have something to hand to act as your tiny silver hammer. I introduced breathing for anxiety, and then, once it became almost second nature, I tried to drink enough water in order to tell my body it's worth being hydrated. Build the tools up slowly as you integrate them into your life.

Slowly integrate different healthy coping mechanisms into your life.

Do *not* take for granted those small taps with your hammer. Do not take for granted each tiny, relentless tap. You can't see it but let me tell you, with every tap you are challenging and weakening the very infrastructure of the ice block. You are compromising and weakening tiny atom by tiny atom. One day, you'll be tapping away and you'll see a crack stretch through the block. Another day, a chunk of ice will clatter to the ground. All the while, slow drips tumble down forming small puddles at your feet. Over time, not overnight.

Your good work is never in vain.

Have you ever learnt a dance routine? You practise the moves over and over so that they become embedded somewhere in the depths of your mind. Then, hopefully, as the music kicks in, you perform the sequence without even thinking about it. It has become so familiar that your body seems to know what it's doing. That's what we're looking for in these techniques.

You didn't start out in life anxious. Your way of coping became a habit that was reinforced through usage.

Don't wait until you feel like you've got the energy to begin to practise these tools.

Hopefully, by now you have a better understanding of the whys, the whats and the hows of your anxiety. The next step is to begin to find healthier ways to respond to your anxious thoughts and form new habits.

Finally, don't wait until you feel like you've got the energy to begin to practise these tools. Don't wait until you suddenly feel motivated. Don't wait until you go through a tough patch or you feel on top of the world. Start today. Pick one and start today. Hopefully the energy, the confident and the positive emotions will come after you've begun to implement the techniques.

I'm hoping that as you begin to persevere, you'll feel proud of yourself as you recognise you're slowly turning that cog in reverse. It might not work every time but you're strengthening a new muscle and you'll get stronger and quicker, and it will feel increasingly natural and instinctive as it becomes a habit.

Setbacks

Setbacks are common and expected when it comes to growth. You might not remember it but the anxiety-coping mechanisms you have will have been instilled at a time of uncertainty and need. They will have been repeated numerous times until they became a reflexive habit. But you're wanting more, you're wanting to instil new coping mechanisms that don't keep you awake at night or send you into anxiety whirlwinds. And that takes time too. You may feel like you're taking a step forward and another couple back, but that's to be expected.

I may be speaking for myself here but many of us are generally impatient beings. It might be that you see development or you conquer a stream of intrusive thoughts. And then, lo and behold, you can't catch a handle on the next batch that come unexpectedly as you sit with a cuppa as the babe naps. Growth can be frustrating. Imagine you bought a packet of dahlia seeds. You've planted them as per the instructions. You watch the soil for a whole day and see no action. It won't grow any faster if you shout at it. Growth is growth and growth takes time.

To work on your anxiety means more than to simply be free from it. It means to grow in awareness and confidence along the way. Keep doing the small things. Keep tapping away with that hammer. If you go through a tough patch, keep tapping. Perhaps what you're doing has helped you not dip as low as you may have. If you go through a good patch and start to feel stronger and more confident . . . don't stop tapping. Often the techniques and the things we do to ground ourselves are the very things helping us.

Fending off anxiety doesn't need to be your only motivation for investing in these tools. These techniques are good habits for life because they will benefit you in so many other ways.

When you work on your anxiety, you grow in awareness and confidence along the way.

I don't 'arrive' at a point where I'm utterly anxiety-free and go, 'WAHOOOOO. *Adios* breathing techniques and imagery! Bye old friends.' Because life takes us through peaks and troughs, unexpected curveballs come our way no matter how prepared we may be. Let the tools you use be the constants in your life, there to support you regardless of how you feel.

Journaling can really aid you in this. Hopefully this book has offered a taster into how helpful it can be. Whilst it might sometimes be hard to see the daily changes, flip back through your writing and you'll get better perspective of how you are moving. Sometimes change is about suddenly realising you've gone a few nights without checking the monitor 229 times. Maybe, one day soon you'll be enjoying an indulgent bath, suddenly realising that a few weeks ago, this would have felt like a worthless waste of time.

I can't promise you, my clients, my kids or myself that our worst fears won't happen. I don't have a crystal ball. But I do promise that if you try to consistently use healthy coping mechanisms and sturdy tools, then the voice of anxiety will get quieter over time.

Keep going. If that ice block hasn't started cracking yet as you've been tapping away, the time will come.

My final words to you

You've reached the end of this book. I acknowledge that it hasn't been a small ask on your time and energy. But I sincerely hope that you feel more equipped and less anxious than when you first opened the pages.

As I've written this, I've done it out of a deep, heartfelt yearning for you to recognise that anxiety doesn't have to be the thief of the joy of these early years of motherhood. It sure is a rollercoaster, with all the phases and stages and sleepless nights, but you deserve more than to be kept awake by intrusive thoughts and overthinking. Or to be bullied by that voice in your mind.

I hope you feel immensely proud of yourself. I know we've probably never met but I can honestly say that I feel proud of every reader that has journeyed through these pages. I know it's not an easy thing to address. It takes bravery, courage and a willingness to pour out precious time and energy on investing in your mental health.

You're not just doing this for you, it is actually hugely selfless. You are doing this for your family too, for your child. You are doing this because they will get so much enjoyment out of seeing you become more yourself. You are taking the time to tackle what may have been generational anxiety that has been passed on through the years. That's an incredibly powerful and generous thing to do.

I encourage you to seek some counselling or therapy if you need it, or even if you simply question whether you do or not. Therapy has been so pertinent in my mental health journey. It often comes with a cost of time, money and energy. However, I promise that prioritising a therapist who is a good fit, above some of the other things that pull on your resource, is a worthy investment.

I hope that you have found more compassion and patience towards yourself. I promise that no matter how messy your feelings, how dark your thoughts, how soap opera-worthy your history, you are deserving of compassion, forgiveness and a chance to feel heard, validated and accepted. I hope that with each act of self-care you engage in, you'll start to realise that those words may have more truth than you have previously led yourself, or been led to believe.

You are deserving of the love and care you give your child.

You are worth the freedom, the life, the possibilities, the deepening relationships and the positive vulnerability that come with not being overwhelmed or hindered by anxiety. You are worth the self-care, the headspace and the support of others. But best of all, you are worthy of accepting the love that comes from your baby.

You are worthy of being their mother.

Anna x

Top Tip

Keep doing the small things.

JOURNAL POINTS

- How do you feel having come to the end of the book?
- Has anything changed for you? If so, what?
- What can you do to keep the momentum up?
- Is there anyone you can share your journey with who can encourage you?

Chapter 13

Emergency pep talks

Here are three pep talks for you to grab in the moments that you need some input.

Panic attack

I know this feels incredibly intense but remember, it's an internal system designed to protect you from physical threat. It has been triggered and that's OK. We're going to use your tools to help it pass. Your mind has run away, your adrenaline is high. It feels like a whirlwind but listen to me. You've been through this before, you've survived, you can do this again. It will be over soon.

Stand or sit with your feet on the ground. Feel the hard, unmoving ground beneath your feet. You are here. Now. This is where life is. This is what's happening. The million possibilities are not real, they are not factual. This is factual – you are here now. Breathe.

Focus on these black and white words on the page. I want you to name five things you can see. List them as if I'm here with you. I want to hear them. OK, now name four things you can touch. Right here in this moment. Now three things you can hear. Nearby, far away, loud, quiet, it doesn't matter. Tell me two things you can smell where you are. Now, finally, one thing you can taste.

Be kind to yourself. Life has shifted so much for you recently. It's going to feel overwhelming sometimes. You're shattered. Your resources are depleted. Now, I want you to ask yourself what you need in this moment. A friendly voice? A hot tea? A hug? Some fresh air? Make it happen. Call someone, step outside, make the drink. You deserve this. You have certainly not failed, you are not weak. You are learning, navigating, making sense of a changed life. And it is good but it is hard, and you are human. Breathe.

I can't do this

From mum to mum I wanted to say – you can do this. I wish I could hop through the page and give you a shoulder massage. You might feel like you can't do this, like you haven't got this, like you want someone to tell you it's all going to be OK. But look, look how far you've come. Look at your little one, look at what you've achieved. You are stronger than you're aware of. You've achieved more than you'll ever give yourself credit for. All those moments before, where you didn't think you could do it, you did. You have. Therefore, you'll do this too. Breathe. Deep, grounding breaths with long exhales. Drop your shoulders.

Is there something you need right now? Emotionally, practically? What step can you take to get that support? Even if it's a tiny step. Maybe it's as simple as a text message. You deserve support, you are not a burden. Think of how it feels when you're able to support a friend. You are simply not created to do this thing called motherhood alone. Might it be that you've been trying to do too much to too high a standard? Is there any corner you can cut, anything that can be deprioritised, anything that can wait for another day or another person?

I've been there and I will be there over and over again. These moments are a human response to what you are going through. Breathe.

Mum guilt

Oh man. Mum guilt. We all feel it but let's unpick it. I know you feel crap right now but you are absolutely no failure. You're a human with limits and man, sometimes they really get pushed in motherhood. We get stretched beyond what we thought possible, in every direction, good and challenging.

There are two types of guilt in my eyes. Let's identify yours. Is it unjustified guilt? Are you feeling guilty because you're shattered and you feel like you've not been inter-acting with your family as you usually do? Perhaps you're unwell, sad, grieving. Perhaps you've not been able to feed as you'd have liked or you feel guilty for the birth you had. This thing you feel guilty about, was it your fault? Did you actively do something wrong? Was it in your control? If a friend came to you saying they felt guilty about this, what would you say?

Some guilt is unjustified. It's not yours to carry because it wasn't your fault that life threw a curveball or something didn't happen as you'd hoped. If you use this guilt to take responsibility where you don't need to, you're using it as a stick to punish yourself with for a crime you didn't commit. This leads to negative self-talk, perhaps self-punishing behaviour. Both things decrease your sense of self-worth. It wasn't your fault. You did the best you could with what you had. Let yourself feel the disappointment, the frustration, the grief and the anger. But please don't use it to shame yourself and beat yourself up.

Is the guilt justified at all? Did you do or say something you wish you hadn't? Well, that guilt isn't there to shame you either. It's there to prompt you, to raise a flag to show you that something needs attention. Perhaps you need to let off steam or research for some tips and techniques so that you might deal with it differently next time. The guilt I feel at using my phone too much around my kids is justified. It's there to prompt me to put in better boundaries, not to make me feel like a horrendous failure of a mum. The guilt I felt a couple of days ago when I shouted at my four-year-old is justified. It's there to prompt me to refresh myself on techniques to calm myself down when things get stressful and I just want to react and join in with his tantrum.

Observe your feeling of guilt. Is it there to prompt you?

What is it trying to prompt you to do? How might you act on that? Or is it perhaps not your guilt to carry. Perhaps you need to take it off your shoulders and let yourself feel the feelings instead. But regardless of the type of guilt you're feeling right now – be kind to yourself. Find some of the grace you offer the people you love because you deserve it too.

Helpful contacts

If you want to take the things you have been exploring in this book further, here are some potential next steps and contacts:

The People-pleasing course

This is a three-week, self-led course addressing people-pleasing, perfectionism, confidence and emotional resilience.

I was a people-pleaser for most of my life until I got sick of being in a cycle of burning-out. I repeatedly gave too much of myself away, leaving only the dregs to keep me going. I knew I didn't want to spend the rest of my life living in a way that was so damaging to my sense of worth and identity. I started a process of addressing this, and as a result, I feel more 'me' than I ever have. I have interwoven my psychological insight and experience as a therapist, along with my personal learning, so that I can gently challenge you on a habit of a lifetime.

See my website (annamathur.com) for a full description and reviews.

NHS and low-cost therapy

Your doctor may be able to refer you for six–twelve sessions of NHS-funded therapy. This might be face-to-face or using an online format. The waiting times and the services are dependent on area.

For low-cost therapy, have a search for services local to you. There might be charities, churches or training institutes that offer no-cost or low-cost sessions for you to access.

Private therapy

The Counselling Directory 'find a therapist' function is my go-to recommendation for finding a therapist. It allows you to search using your postcode and browse the profiles of therapists in your area.

NHS website

The NHS website is a brilliant resource for learning about all things mental and physical on health. It offers advice on where to seek support and other next steps you might like to take in addressing any symptoms.

Supportive websites based in the UK

Anxietyuk.org.uk
Mind.org.uk
Nopanic.org.uk
NCT.org.uk
Maternalmentalhealthalliance.org

Telephone helplines (UK)

Pandas Foundation (prenatal, antenatal and postnatal mental
health support line): 0843 289 8401
Samaritans: 116 123
SANEline: 0300 304 7000

Acknowledgements

Lauren, my wonderful literary agent. You popped into my inbox as if you knew that my heart was full of words that needed to be written. I couldn't have found a better fit or kinder person to guide me through what has been an entirely new experience. You helped me weather the storm of disappointment through the sturdy hope you held. We did it! We did it!

Jill, my editor, when I walked away from our first meeting together, the first thing I said was 'I hope she picks me'. I knew you got me, my heart, my passion and my vision for this book, and I so hoped you would be the one to bring it to fruition. Thank you for taking a chance on me. You are a skilled and lovely editor, and I feel honoured to work with you. I hope to make you proud.

To my wonderful friends who have cheer-led this whole process. Who have been on the receiving end of texts and calls, and requests for title ideas and read-throughs: Hannah W, Marianna, Hannah F, Kathryn, Sophie, Jo, Sasha, Sarah, Laura, Kate, Rachel, Coley, Elle and Sally.

To Ella who loves my kids almost as much as I do. You

have cared for them so beautifully whilst I write. And for Jenny and Satish, my brilliant in-laws. You are forever interested in my work and proud of me. It means the world. Thank you for stepping in to help with the kids so many times.

Deborah my therapist. It's been so good to re-engage with you after five years! It always astounds me how much you remember of the words I uttered years ago. Your insight has been invaluable. I know you really see me. Thank you for your emotional support throughout this process.

Mum, I am sure that it is because of your input and guidance throughout my life that I have such a deep passion and compassion for people. You have taught me to look further beyond what I first encounter. You have faithfully helped me untangle endless complex circumstances and emotions. You have always been there, patiently waiting in the wings through the difficult times even though it must have been so hard to see me struggle. You were ready for the moment I was ready. You share my vision for this book because our hearts beat for the same stuff – that people will feel hope.

Oscar, you made me a mum. Your sweet, sensitive soul has been so gracious as I've fumbled my way through learning what it means to be a mother. You taught me that I was ultimately loveable, for if you could love me so wholeheartedly, then maybe I could love me too. Charlie, we had a tough first year. You led me to the very ends of myself and showed me quite how strong and capable I could be. You turned me into a lioness and you make me laugh with your heavenly quirks. Florence, you're the cherry on my cupcake and a healing balm for what has gone before. You three are my reasons. You are my motivation that this book will enable other mums to realise their worth within and beyond motherhood, in the way you've led me to realising mine.

To my husband, Tarun. You are one of a kind. Without you, your support and your unwavering belief in me, there wouldn't be a book. And without your solid and persistent love, my journey wouldn't have been one that could hopefully shape the course of others. You loved me at my most broken, which is fab, because I will always be a little broken. But I'm increasingly OK with that, because I was always enough for you.

Index

Note: page numbers in *italics* refer to illustrations.